For a Child's Sake

For a Child's Sake

History of The Children's Hospital, Denver, Colorado, 1910–1990

Rickey Hendricks and Mark S. Foster

University Press of Colorado

© 1994 by the University Press of Colorado
P.O. Box 849
Niwot, Colorado 80544

The University Press of Colorado is a cooperative publishing enterprise supported, in part, by Adams State College, Colorado State University, Fort Lewis College, Mesa State College, Metropolitan State College of Denver, University of Colorado, University of Northern Colorado, University of Southern Colorado, and Western State College of Colorado.

Library of Congress Cataloging-in-Publication Data

Hendricks, Rickey Lynn.
    For a child's sake: history of the Children's Hospital, Denver,
  Colorado, 1910–1990 / Rickey Hendricks and Mark S. Foster.
        p. cm.
    Includes index.
    ISBN 0-87081-349-8
    1. Children's Hospital (Denver, Colo.) — History. 2. Children —
  Hospitals — Colorado — Denver — History. I. Foster, Mark S. II.
  Title.
  RJ28.D46H46 1994
  382.1'9892'000978883 —dc20   94-19209
                                                           CIP

The paper used in this publication meets the minimum requirements of the American National Standard for Information Sciences — Permanence of Paper for Printed Library Materials. ANSI Z39.48–1984

∞

10 9 8 7 6 5 4 3 2 1

The Children's Hospital Association and its board of directors are pleased to dedicate this book to the many young people who, at a unique and significant moment in their lives, were patients at The Children's Hospital of Denver.

Contents

Foreword

Today I had lively telephone visits with three individuals who live in Denver and were patients at The Children's Hospital. Mary Jean Nicely is eighty-one years old; Edgar Biggs Sheldon is seventy-six; Derry "Rooster" Felton is ten years old and was discharged last week, having sacrificed his angry appendix to the cause of science.

These three people don't know one another but as patients they share a common bond. Mary Jean and Edgar were hospitalized in the small rooms of the remodeled brownstone residence at 2221 Downing that had, with moderate but exultant fanfare, opened its doors to "the sick babies and little ones of Denver" on February 17, 1910. Oca Cushman, R.N. and first superintendent, who at the time began a disciplined love affair with The Children's Hospital that lasted nearly fifty years, led the first patients inside.

When a cavalcade of "motor cars," with their exhausts billowing in the clear frigid air of February 12, 1917, and "a dozen doctors" arrived to transport the entire patient population of thirty from the quickly outgrown facility to the gleaming new hospital at Nineteenth Avenue and Downing Street, Mary Jean and Edgar were among those present. Mary Jean was flat on her back with tuberculosis of the spine; Edgar had his hands restrained to keep him from digging at his severe generalized eczema.

Mary Jean remembers the trip well. She was wrapped in blankets, and Dr. John Amesse carried her out to the car because he was her pediatrician. Edgar's memories of the long-awaited move are distillations of what he was told by his parents when he was older. "And Doc," he told me over the phone, "my eczema never really did go away."

Derry's recollections are as crisp as yesterday's newspaper, intensified by discomfort and the threat of the unknown, but softened by caring hands. I asked him about the food. "It was OK," he proclaimed, "but my mom's is better." (So much for hospital cuisine!) "The nurses were nice; one of them looks like my aunt who lives in Des Moines."

The kaleidoscopic events taking place between the hospitalizations of these three children — the unpredictable and implacable march of eighty years — constitute almost the entire life of The Children's Hospital. Herodotus argued that he wrote of the ancient Greeks to secure for them "the honor of remembrance." The Children's Hospital of today is steadfastly going about the heady business of creating its own past: "glimmers in the misty great seas of recollection."

The board of directors intend, by means of these chapters, to secure remembrance for the hospital, its patients, and the individuals beyond counting who were part of the dynamic and engrossing years before the final decade of the twentieth century. As the armature of fact was fleshed out by the authors, with the guidance of The Children's Hospital Historical Society and an intimidating room full of meticulously kept records, the hospital became personalized and the work became an intimate biography.

When those two resilient pioneers in the life of The Children's Hospital, Mrs. George B. Packard[1] and Dr. John Amesse,[2] reflected in print on the hospital of their time and place, they had it easy in a sense. The abrasive spectrum of childhood illness was no less threatening than it is today but was of a vastly different nature. In most instances the treatment of a hospitalized child was largely compassionate nursing care and the generalized affection that had become the hospital's hallmark, carried on against a backdrop of numerous nonspecific treatment maneuvers. The reputation of The Children's Hospital nursing staff and the fierce allegiance of its volunteers and support staff were legendary — and still are.

By the mid-1940s, energized by the stunning development of antibiotic therapy, made-to-measure biochemical breakthroughs, undreamt-of technologic progress, and sociologic pressures, the character of The Children's Hospital was forced to change. For decades successive boards of directors, assisted considerably by the Tammen and Boettcher families and other devoted benefactors, had charted the course of a relatively uncomplicated organization — a "cottage industry." They all dealt with many of the vexing problems that face health care institutions today. They wrestled then as now with the conviction that every child should have undreamt-of access to health care — but just what was to be provided? And how was it to be done? By whom? And who would pay for it? Circumstances haven't changed much; the same decisions are being agonized over and must be resolved today and tomorrow, but the magnitude of the contemporary responsibility is a fierce challenge.

Ethical and moral dilemmas that were unheard of in those early days when physicians often made house calls in a buggy, on a number 10 yellow streetcar, or in a Model-U light six Stevens-Duryea, have proliferated to distort reality and defy rational thought. The incubus of medical-legal jeopardy stands as a bedside companion to any of those who bear responsibility. The Children's Hospital of today, "circling the wagons" in its continuing effort to carry out the mission forthrightly stated by its founders more than eighty years ago, would be unrecognizable to Mrs. George Packard, Hattie Colburn, or Dr. Minnie C.T. Love.

There is a problem inherent in any effort to tell the story of an enterprise as complex and personal as The Children's Hospital, looking back over so many years. A multitude of unique and talented people were vitally involved in one way or another. We have chosen to name a few as prototypes of the many. Those highlighted in the history bear a distinct responsibility, for they represent others who, in critical periods of the institution's growth, served The Children's Hospital with superlative loyalty and dedication — "for a child's sake"! This book seeks to secure for them, for all the patients they served across the tumultuous years, and for the hospital they molded into one of the finest children's hospitals in the country, the honor of remembrance.

Seymour E. Wheelock, M.D.
October 1993

Notes

1. Mrs. George Packard, Sr., *A Little Story of The Children's Hospital of Denver*, 1934.
2. John W. Amesse, M.D., *History of The Children's Hospital of Denver, 1910–1947* (Denver: The Children's Hospital Association, 1947).

Acknowledgments

The Children's Hospital Association gratefully acknowledges the members of The Children's Hospital Historical Society for their tireless efforts in perpetuating the history of the hospital. The members are: Jeaneene F. Anderson, William Bailey, M.D., L. Joseph Butterfield, M.D., Janet Cunningham, R.N., C. Richard Hawes, M.D., Ann Klenk, Winifred R. Moss, Walter S. Rosenberry III, Lou Shannon, James K. Todd, M.D., Seymour Wheelock, M.D., and Harry Wilson, M.D.

Photography Credits

Cover	Phil LaRocco
Bertha Rich teaching class	Rocky Mountain Photo Company
Tammen Hall	Mile High Photo Company
Lula Lubchenco	Seymour E. Wheelock, M.D.
Santa Claus	*Denver Post*
Oca Cushman Wing	Yuji Oishi, M.D.
Charlene Holton, M.D.	Bob Scott
L. J. Butterfield, M.D.	Bob Scott
Newborn Center scenery	Tom Masamori
Ann Kosloske, M.D.r	Gary Guisinge
Billy Parkin	Michael Gamer
J. H. Silversmith, Jr.	Berkeley-Lainson-Denver
Elliott Stacey	Michael Gamer

Children's Hospital Photographers

Jim Barbour	Yuji Oishi, M.D.
Tia Brayman	George Silver
David Chavez	Ivey S. Stevens
Steve Kast	

Photographs, if not specifically credited, are from The Children's Hospital Collection.

The Children's Hospital Historical Society owes much to the many groups and individuals whose knowledge and interest in The Children's Hospital over the years has provided colorful substance to the tapestries of the hospital's eight decades of service to the region.

Although the history of The Children's Hospital has been written by professional historians, there was a small group of individuals who devoted many hours of hard work and the benefits of their knowledge of the institution to make the dream of *For a Child's Sake* possible.

The members affectionately recognize the role of Winifred R. Moss, who served as liaison between the authors, the hospital, and the members of the historical society. She brought to this complicated project the same genial but persistent momentum and precision that marked her twenty years as executive secretary to the board of directors.

Walter S. Rosenberry III, Chairman
Jeaneene F. Anderson
William Carl Bailey, M.D.
L. Joseph Butterfield, M.D.
Janet C. Cunningham, R.N., M.S.
C. Richard Hawes, M.D.
Ann Klenk
Lou Shannon
James K. Todd, M.D.
Seymour E. Wheelock, M.D.
Harry Wilson, M.D.

Chapter 1

In the Beginning

In his annual report of 1877 the first Colorado State Board of Health president, physician Frederick J. Bancroft, claimed that the whole world sought the "benefits our famed climate can dispense to those seeking restoration to health and strength." Denver's children were the objects of this boast. According to Bancroft, Colorado's health providers would seek "to ascertain in what localities and at what altitude the growing child may gain the best physical and mental development. If high altitude increased the breathing capacity and strength of the heart, and the plains produce tall, athletic men, it is not improbable that places may be found in Colorado where growing children may attain best possible health and longevity."[1] The democratic frontier spirit was nurtured in the pioneer family and embodied, metaphorically, by the westering child. While partially rooted in Old World and eastern traditions and precedents, health care for children in the western United States would take on its own distinctive character.

Before the eighteenth-century Enlightenment, European hospitals were charitable charnel houses; child mortality rates often approached 90 or even 100 percent. They offered shelter for the sick rather than scientific improvement of particular ailments. Yet Enlightenment attitudes affected hospitals, which began to incorporate medical training, research, and healing for the needy sick in a nurturing, clean environment. Newly conceived and rapidly developing awareness of special needs of children symbolized hope for improved lives for all citizens of the free state. As historian Philippe Aries demonstrated, in previous centuries children were perceived of and treated as miniature adults. The first outpatient dispensary exclusively for sick children was established by George Armstrong in London in 1769, but it closed in 1782 "for lack of public interest and support." It served 35,000 children during its thirteen-year existence. Its immediate successor was London's Royal Infirmary for Children.[2]

The first recognizable children's hospital on the European continent was the Hospital des Enfants Malades in Paris, founded in 1802. At the outset it appeared as a great reform, saving sick children from despicable conditions at the Hotel Dieu, where they were placed eight in a bed, indiscriminately mixed with adults with infectious diseases of every type. One historian claims, however, that ambitious physicians corrupted the purpose of the Hospital des Enfants. The large number of patients facing almost certain death provided the prestigious "clinical/pathological Paris School" with experimental subjects for the scientific study of childhood illnesses.[3]

In 1800 there were only two hospitals for the sick in the nation. The few hospitals that existed in early nineteenth-century America were located in teeming, urban port cities as a means of social control. They treated transient populations of seamen, soldiers, merchant travelers, new immigrants, the "deserving poor," and young workers moving in increasing numbers from farm to city without support from a kinship network. The Marine Hospital Corps for seamen was set up in 1798 as the first federal health program, with a hospital in New York. (The Marine Hospital Corps was made the U.S. Public Health Service in 1912.) Elite trustees and caregivers acted according to religious tenets of benevolence and a "stewardship of wealth" but offered little or no hope for physical improvement. Scions of the upper classes found themselves in such institutions only in unfortunate cases of accident while far from home or in cases of hopeless insanity.

Science and male physicians were minuscule parts of the nineteenth-century U.S. hospital. Florence Nightingale's precepts for nurses' training and moral order in the hospital setting challenged the primacy of medical science and influence of physicians on nineteenth-century institutional development. Nightingale's *Notes on Hospitals* in 1859 integrated a sanitary code for hospital construction, administration, and patient care. Lack of cleanliness, sanitation, and careful procedures to air and fumigate the abodes of the poorer urban classes was viewed as either a fatal moral lapse or ignorance. Nurses created the conditions; thus Nightingale considered the nurse's role essentially spiritual and central to the hospital's healing mission. Patients spent months in "convalescence," even doing their own cooking and cleaning in a kind of boardinghouse arrangement where nutrition, cleanliness, and nursing were the primary tools for allowing nature, not medicine, to take its course.[4]

Female philanthropists and staff dominated the earliest U.S. hospitals for children. The first hospitals for children in this country were the

Nursery and Child's Hospital in New York City, founded in 1854 as a nursery for the children of wet nurses and other working mothers, and Children's Hospital of Philadelphia, founded in 1855. The Chicago Hospital for Women and Children opened in 1865, and both Boston Children's Hospital and the New York Foundling Asylum in 1869. Through the 1870s hospitals for children were still concentrated on the East Coast.

Typical children's hospitals of the 1860s and 1870s were private institutions in converted family residences, housing only about twenty patients. Supporters included trustees who gave financial support, visiting ladies, and outside physicians, all working on a minimal budget. Some hospitals had full-time matrons providing custodial care, but most caretaking was by volunteer lady visitors. As hospitals evolved in succeeding decades, they added paid nurses, consulting physician boards, and salaried resident physicians. Almost all such institutions were charitable, patronized almost exclusively by the poor.

Boston Children's Hospital typified these early pediatric institutions. According to one historian, although the hospital's primary mission was "medical and surgical treatment of the diseases of children," its early annual reports stressed routine nurturing rather than medical activities. It clearly was established for innocent victims of poverty and urban squalor; patients were called "the little waifs who crowd our poorer streets." Physicians took on hospital posts out of a sense of noblesse oblige to these children, but also because hospitals and foundling homes gave them experience in treating children's diseases. Pediatrics evolved much more slowly than other formally recognized specialties. The American Medical Association was created in 1847; the AMA Section of Diseases of Children formed in 1881, and the American Pediatric Society in 1888.[5]

In the West female physicians played a primary role in a more egalitarian environment. The western frontier presented new opportunities for physicians of both sexes. The California and Colorado goldfields drew physicians in unusual numbers. Many prominent families came to Colorado seeking a cure for tuberculosis, along with thousands who could afford only minimal care in hastily constructed tent clinics and sanitoria. Several of these pioneer families produced offspring who later played prominent roles in founding or staffing Children's Hospital. For many years after the founding of Denver in 1859, promoters such as Henry H. Tammen and Stanley Wood claimed in *The Great Divide* and other periodicals that robust health emanated from the natural purity of Colorado's high country. In fact, Denver and the mining towns of the region suffered crowding, environmental pollution, and faulty municipal sanitation, the same problems found in older eastern cities.

Historian Elliott West has observed that in the sparsely settled West, children took on intense significance to the overwhelmingly male population of early mining and supply towns. Child welfare assumed crucial importance in regions where children were rare. In retrospect it is clear that many pioneers abused the natural environment, exacerbating health hazards. Contagious diseases were easily passed from one wagon train to another. In campsites careless disposal of human waste and other thoughtless acts spelled danger for later arrivals. During westward migrations sickness was the number-one killer, more prevalent than starvation, exposure, and accidents combined. Children were more vulnerable than adults because they had not had all childhood diseases and had developed fewer immunities.[6]

Thus although medical care was imperative from Denver's earliest days, actual services emerged very gradually. Levi J. Russell of Georgia was the first physician to come to Colorado, but he was far more interested in making money than healing the sick. Russell arrived with two brothers in June 1858 to pan gold in Cherry Creek, and they built the first cabin at the Auraria townsite. They made one of the first big strikes at Russell Gulch near Central City.

The few women in the gold camps probably did more to sustain community health than gold-seeking male doctors. Early hospitals reflected the democracy of the territorial society. For a time Clara Brown, a black woman, ran a hospital in her home in Central City.[7] Perhaps there were too few women and established philanthropists to provide sufficient moral and economic support for basic human services in the early mining camps. Certainly the overwhelming majority of adult males were too busy to pay attention to matters that did not involve either making money or relaxation. Sickness and disease festered in the mining camps because of ignorance, indifference, and poor sanitation. Inhabitants lived with rotting animals and waste, impure drinking water, and air filled with dust from mechanized drilling and smelting operations.

Denverites fared better than mining town inhabitants at higher elevations. City builders, concerned about the Queen City's public image, emphasized healthfulness of the natural environment and the benefits of progressive city life. Early hospitals in Denver were started by a fledgling medical establishment. In 1860 several doctors founded the Jefferson Medical Society, along with Denver City Hospital, a semipublic log building at Sixteenth and Blake. There were other efforts in the 1860s to care for the indigent sick who were lodged in Denver's poorhouse and private homes for fees paid by the county. The poorhouse was located initially at Eleventh Street between Wazee and Market, later at Ninth and Champa. In 1873 a large brick building was constructed at Sixth and Cherokee as a combination poorhouse and hospital. In an 1874 report the county hospital listed 189 patients; eighteen had apparently died in the hospital over the preceding twelve months.[8]

Private efforts to provide health care emerged simultaneously. In 1873 St. Vincent's Hospital, sponsored by the Sisters of Charity of Leavenworth, Kansas, opened at 1421 Arapahoe Street. It moved to Twenty-sixth and Market shortly thereafter, followed by yet another move in 1876 to a building at Eighteenth and Humboldt. In 1876 its name was changed to Saint Joseph's Hospital. The hospital basically served working-class Catholics. St. Luke's Hospital, a two-story wooden, converted hotel with twenty-one rooms just off Federal Boulevard, was founded by Episcopalians in the early 1880s. To avoid problems of its "suburban location," such as doctors having to travel through the city "bottoms" at night, a new building was constructed at Nineteenth and Pennsylvania in 1891. St. Luke's later affiliated with Presbyterian Hospital. St. Anthony's was organized by the Sisters of St. Francis in 1893 and located off Federal Boulevard at Cheltenham Avenue between Eighteenth and Nineteenth Avenues. St. Anthony's was connected to the city by an electric streetcar line; construction was completed in 1894. In 1901 its four-story brick building with 211 beds was staffed by thirty-six part-time private physicians and forty nuns.[9]

Early Denver pioneer doctors, nurses, and other female reformers laid the groundwork for developing a children's hospital that merged the medical knowledge and social mission of their predecessors in the eastern communities from which they came. In eastern hospitals, lay trustees exercised a stewardship of wealth, defined by the philanthropic urban upper class. Victorian reformers adopted the prevalent sentimental attitude toward children and family that replaced the seventeenth-century belief that children replicated the sins of their parents, with their value based primarily on their potential economic contribution to family survival. In the West an optimistic view of the child and community replaced the perceived need to control the rough and disorderly industrial population in eastern cities.

By the last decades of the century, physicians applying new medical discoveries began to reshape the hospital from a charitable social institution to one that incorporated the latest scientific techniques. The predominantly male physicians superimposed scientific imperatives upon Nightingale's formula for moral order, ultimately winning authority inside hospital walls. But the dichotomy between "sympathy and science," the domestic and medical science spheres, created continuing tensions between the male and female professionals in the evolution of early children's hospitals. Organizers sought to merge nurturing and order with advanced medical knowledge and application of scientific methods. Methods of artificial infant feeding became a major research focus. Doctors, mothers, and women managers all recognized that inadequate feeding of sick and abandoned infants triggered a high mortality rate among poor babies. Physicians, mostly male, who specialized in infant feeding joined with urban female social activists in a nationwide pure milk campaign, creating milk stations and developing artificial formulas. In fact, modern pediatrics basically emerged from infant feeding concerns. Middle- and upper-class mothers welcomed "scientific" nutrition for their children, and they in turn sought to educate indigent and working-class mothers.[10]

Pediatricians and reformers campaigned for public hygiene and pure milk programs through strict sanitation codes for dairies and urban milk stations that offered either free or very inexpensive sterilized milk. The first "milk depots" in street-level booths or storefronts were set up in New York tenement districts during the early 1890s. From the turn of the century until World War I, maternal and child welfare reform focused on child labor, tainted food, and educating mothers about infant feeding and hygiene.[11]

As the frontier became more settled, Colorado's women and physicians were increasingly active in the national crusade for child health and welfare. By 1890 Denver's population of 106,713 still had no hospital just for children;[12] however, individuals who would play central roles in founding Children's Hospital were gathering in Denver. Colorado's first specialist in pediatric orthopaedics, Dr. George B. Packard, Sr., was born in 1852 on a farm in Jericho Center, Vermont. He received his M.D. degree from the University of Vermont Medical College in 1874 and began postgraduate study in orthopaedics at the Medical College of New York. By 1880 Packard had a private practice in Hartford, Connecticut. In 1887 he became a charter

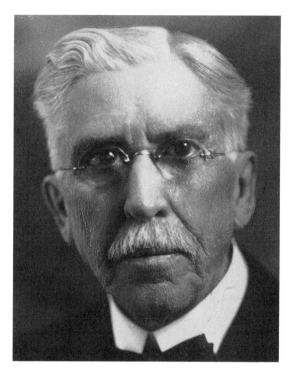

Dr. George B. Packard, Sr., pioneer surgeon and orthopae-
dist in Denver, was one of the founders and first president
of the hospital's medical and surgical staff.

member of the American Orthopaedic Association, and presented the first
paper at that association. A year later, seriously ill with tuberculosis, he
moved to Colorado Springs. When his health had improved, he moved his
family to Denver in 1890 and resumed full-time practice in orthopaedics.
In 1892 he was appointed professor of orthopaedic surgery at the University of Colorado School of Medicine.[13]

Three other eastern-trained physicians eventually comprised the first
medical staff at The Children's Hospital. Herbert B. Whitney was born in
1856 and received a B.S., followed by an M.D. degree in 1882 from Harvard
and two years of postgraduate study in Europe. He began practice in
Boston but, like Packard, went to Colorado to "chase the cure" for tuberculosis. After recovering in Salida, he moved to Denver in 1887, where he
became professor of children's diseases at the University of Colorado

8

For a Child's Sake

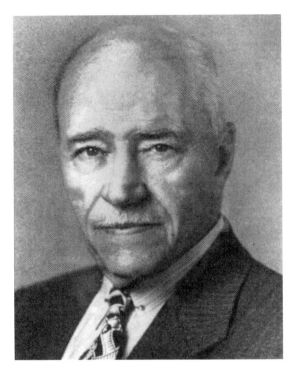

Dr. John W. Amesse, author of *History of The Children's Hospital of Denver, 1910–1947*, and private practicing staff pediatrician for almost fifty years.

School of Medicine and later professor of medicine at Gross Medical College. By 1922 he was credited with forty-six publications.[14]

John W. Amesse was born in 1874 of French Canadian parents. His M.D. degree was from the University of Michigan in 1898. As a member of the Marine Hospital Corps (now the U.S. Public Health Service), within a ten-year period he served in San Francisco during the plague outbreak of 1900; as a quarantine officer in the Philippines; as an immigration officer in Seattle, Honolulu, and on Ellis Island; in the New Orleans yellow fever epidemic; in the Marine Hospital in Illinois; and finally as a special government representative in Costa Rica. In 1910–1911 he studied pediatrics at Johns Hopkins and Bellevue. He then moved to Denver, where he joined the CU medical faculty.

Franklin P. Gengenbach was born in 1875 in Philadelphia and received his M.D. degree from the University of Pennsylvania in 1899. He did

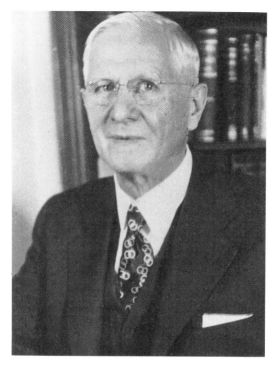

Dr. Franklin P. Gengenbach, referred to as the "Father of
Colorado pediatrics," was the first physician in this area
to limit his practice to pediatrics. He and his contempo-
raries were designated on the hospital medical staff as
"infant feeders" for many years.

graduate work in Berlin and Vienna in 1915, then entered private practice
in Denver as the city's first full-time pediatrician. Later he headed the
Department of Pediatrics at the University of Colorado Medical School and
was a founder of the American Academy of Pediatrics and the American
Board of Pediatrics. Widely respected as a regional consultant in his specialty, he also founded the Rocky Mountain Pediatric Society.[15]

The Rocky Mountain region also provided some opportunities for
professional women who eventually made significant contributions to
Children's Hospital. The Colorado Medical Association refused women in
the 1870s, but a decade later the Denver Medical Association accepted
them. Dr. Mary H.B. Bates, a graduate of the Women's Medical College of
Philadelphia, arrived in Leadville with the silver boom in 1878. Two years

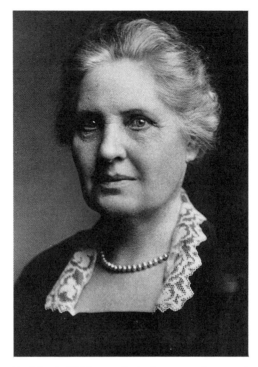

Dr. Minnie C.T. Love, who had temporarily opened
a summer "tent hospital" for children "of the poor"
in 1897, originally conceived the idea of a Denver
hospital for children and campaigned successfully
for the hospital at 2221 Downing Street.

later she went to Denver, where she served in public health for the next
thirty years. She pioneered Colorado's public school health law, considered
a national model in the early twentieth century.[16]

Minnehaha Cecelia Francesca Tucker Love was born in 1856 at La
Crosse, Wisconsin, but the family moved to Washington, D.C. Her mother
was a daughter of Nelson Roosevelt, a distant relative of a future president,
Theodore Roosevelt. Minnie was admitted to Howard University as one of
the first white women to study medicine there. After graduation and
marriage she moved with her husband, Charles C. Love, to San Francisco
and began her first practice there. In 1891 the Loves spent time in London,
where she did postgraduate work in obstetrics and children's diseases —
the only specialties open to women. The couple then settled in Denver,

where Charles Love was assistant treasurer of the Colorado Supply Company until his early death from tuberculosis in 1906.[17]

Dr. Love enthusiastically entered the lists of social activists among professional and middle-class women of Denver. She became a suffragist and an avid member of several local women's and professional associations. Her professional ties included the state and county medical society affiliates of the American Medical Association. She was the first woman appointed to the State Board of Charities and Corrections and helped establish the State Industrial School for Girls.

Nursing provided another career opportunity for women. Oca Rush lived in Pittsville, Missouri, and attended the state college at Warrensburg.[18] In 1889 she visited Denver, where she met high school teacher A. J. Cushman. They married on July 31, 1890; he died in 1895. Oca Cushman lived with her sister until 1900, but desiring a career, at age thirty she entered nurse training at St. Luke's Hospital in Denver. She was an older applicant but met the moral standard and other requirements.

There were several local training schools for nurses in the late nineteenth century. Not until 1905 did nursing require state licensing, and it is unknown how many of the 600 nurses and midwives listed in Denver's 1900 census had any formal training. But many opportunities existed for the young woman committed to health care, including St. Joseph's Hospital and St. Luke's; the latter opened a nursing school in 1892. The Colorado Training School for Nurses began courses in 1887.[19]

In Colorado, women's participation in politics was circumscribed. Denver's middle- and upper-class women helped working-class women and children through voluntary clubs and charities rather than political reform. The Women's Christian Temperance Union established a day nursery in 1888 for working mothers and opened Colorado Cottage Home for unwed mothers. The Young Women's Christian Association crusaded against child labor and gave food and shelter to the homeless. In 1894 the *Rocky Mountain News* reported that Denver was a "city of women's clubs." The Denver Women's Club sponsored community vegetable gardens to feed the poor, supported a tent hospital for children near City Park, and in 1895 backed creation of the State Home for Dependent Children. Colorado granted women's suffrage in 1893, the first state to do so by male popular vote (Wyoming gave women the vote sooner, but by a constitutional mandate). Colorado suffragists included Drs. Minnie Love and Mary B. Bates, along with 10,000 other women.[20]

By the late 1890s most of the critical ingredients and personalities vital
to the establishment of Children's Hospital had arrived in the Queen City.
In the summer of 1897 Dr. Love received support of the Denver Women's
Club and other society matrons to start an outdoor tent hospital at Eighteenth and Gaylord Streets for infants and children suffering from gastrointestinal disorders. It was not an original concept. Earlier the Boston
Children's Hospital and Chicago Memorial Hospital had sponsored outdoor summer "hospitals," which implemented theories of the therapeutic
value of fresh air and ventilation. In the pre-antibiotic era these were the
only known weapons against serious infant illness and mortality from
diarrhea and dehydration. Chicago also had the Lincoln Park Sanitarium,
an open-air day camp for infants.

Thanks to her professional connections, Dr. Love had access to many
contemporary ideas about children's hospitals. She was also probably well
aware of potential pitfalls as well as problems encountered by earlier
institutions caring for children. At Chicago Memorial Hospital the female
board of managers and male medical staff diverged sharply in the mid–
1890s over social versus medical roles of the hospital. Physicians sought
expansion to house more of the 10,000 homeless children, many of whom
were sick. The managers opposed hospitalization of sick infants because of
the high institutional mortality rate. Infant care distorted the mortality rate
of the hospital as a whole and created a pessimistic environment that
hampered recovery of the older children. Disputes between the women
managers and male physicians of Chicago eventually caused an irreparable
philosophical rift. Similar conflicts over perceived missions eventually
divided doctors and managers at Boston Infant's Hospital in the 1880s.[21]

Denver women lauded the region's best curative geographic features
— its wide open spaces, high country "ventilation," and salubrious arid
climate. In early May 1897 the *Rocky Mountain News* listed the directors of
the Babies' Summer Hospital, who held an "enthusiastic meeting" at the
home of Mrs. Jasper D. Ward. The women obtained free service from the
electric light and water companies and bedding supplies from other
sources. The women of St. Barnabas Church donated nightgowns. The
Women's Club held a sewing bee to "make up" the material donated to the
hospital. The tent hospital, with six nurses, could accommodate fifty children up to the age of five.

In June 1897 the *News* reported "two rows of weather-beaten tents"
and pictured a happy bucolic scene of "little invalids running around the

enclosure, rolling in the alfalfa, and shouting in glee over their freedom."
Uniforms and visual images were important. "The nurses, daintily attired
in summer dresses, with little white caps, move to and fro, sometimes
exercising a feeble infant in a carriage, at other times giving chase to some
unruly youngster who proudly calls the attention of the passer-by to his
brand new sky-blue overalls." Newspapers proclaimed that the sick underprivileged children of Denver thrived in this environment. The happy
"unruly youngster . . . scampers madly around the inclosure with the
good-natured nurse in pursuit," a picture of the late Victorian idyllic,
affectionate view of childhood.

Denver's lady philanthropists valued favorable publicity for their
ambitious undertaking. As they looked toward the next century, they
sensed that caring for Denver's sick children would be an increasingly
expensive and professionalized community endeavor. Newspaper report-
ers deliberately assisted the women's public relations campaign. The overall scene was carefully composed, like a French romantic painting, with
nurses and children alike well regimented. One reporter wrote, "The nurses
are assiduous to the little patients, who for the most part are perfectly
obedient and accept whatever comes their way without demurring." The
physicians were firmly in control, the nurses congenial and helpful. "Physicians in charge are seen daily visiting their charges, and overseeing the
premises" while "everyone is shown over the premises by the attentive
nurses." Good order and nutrition were emphasized, sometimes in saccha-
rine terms. In the dining tent "the little boys and girls . . . with beaming
faces [sit] expectantly. . . . Like Jack Spratt and his wife, they leave the
platter clean."[22]

These idyllic scenes were in vivid contrast to a quite different scene
of urban disorder depicted by the president of the State Board of Health at
the turn of the century. Epidemics of smallpox, diphtheria, typhoid, and
cholera plagued residents in Denver, allegedly the "filthiest city in the
United States." He blamed "foul air, soil sodden with filth from cess pools
and privies, and polluted water," much like the well-worn trail west to the
goldfields a generation earlier. National Jewish Hospital housed some of
the children with tuberculosis, who were part of the one-fifth to one-third
of the state population afflicted. Infant mortality reached 10 percent of live
births.[23]

The tent hospital apparently continued for a second summer in 1898
but was closed, perhaps because of pressures for volunteer efforts support-

ing the Spanish American War. Many doctors serving the tent hospital also had strong commitments to public health, serving on various state boards and commissions. Dr. Love, for example, assisted the Red Cross and continued her professional and public service activities for several decades. She was even elected to the Colorado Assembly for one term, 1926–1928, and as a state representative sponsored a bill requiring unwed mothers to breast-feed their babies.[24]

Fifty years ago research and publication were already important for those seeking recognition and advancement in pediatrics. Dr. Love, who died in 1942, was particularly effective at the initial creative stage of institution-building. Her obituary, though meant to be flattering, revealed the double standard used in evaluating professional women of her generation. Lauding her as an incorporator and lifelong member of The Children's Hospital Association, the somewhat patronizing eulogy stressed her feminine attributes: "A handsome woman, with a ringing voice and a gift of sound logic, she could speak [out on] any cause she espoused to success and at the same time never failed to recognize the value of being completely feminine."[25] Though some female colleagues sought full acceptance by the male medical establishment, she chose another sphere of influence: addressing the larger concerns of women, children, and family in her new western community. Her path clearly diverged from the male domain of medical research and academia.

The lay female founders of the nation's first children's hospitals stressed charity rather than science. In the vanguard of the army of Progressive urban reformers mobilizing the nation to meet the challenges of the twentieth century, they sought to ameliorate the growth pains of rapid industrialization and urban expansion.

Notes

1. F. J. Bancroft, M.D., "President's Address, Colorado State Board of Health," *First Annual Report* (Denver: *Rocky Mountain News* Steam Printing House, 1877), 17, 19.

2. Philippe Aries, *Centuries of Childhood: A Social History of Family Life* (New York: A. A. Knopf, 1962); Eduard Seidler, "An Historical Survey of Children's Hospitals," in Lindsay Granshaw and Roy Porter, eds., *The Hospital in History* (London and New York: Routledge, 1989), 181–184.

3. Granshaw and Porter, *The Hospital in History*, 181–197; quotation, 187.

4. Charles E. Rosenberg, *The Care of Strangers: The Rise of America's Hospital System* (New York: Basic Books, Inc., 1987), 18–19, 128–135.

5. Boston Children's Hospital, *Annual Report for 1871*, quoted in Morris J. Vogel, *The Invention of the Modern Hospital, Boston 1870–1930* (Chicago: University of Chicago Press, 1980), 23;

Sydney A. Halpern, *American Pediatrics: The Social Dynamics of Professionalism, 1880–1980* (Berkeley: University of California Press, 1988), 40–47, 178n.

6. Elliott West, *Growing Up With the Country: Childhood on the Far Western Frontier* (Albuquerque: University of New Mexico Press, 1989).

7. Richard J. Shikes, M.D., *Rocky Mountain Medicine: Doctors, Drugs, and Disease in Early Colorado* (Boulder: Johnson Publishing Co., 1986), 33, 34.

8. Ibid., 57–59.

9. Ibid., 66–68.

10. Rickey Hendricks, "Feminism and Maternalism in Early Hospitals for Children: San Francisco and Denver, 1875–1915," *Journal of the West* 32 (July 1993): 61–69. Sources for these trends include Regina Morantz-Sanchez, *Sympathy and Science: Women Physicians in American Medicine* (New York: Oxford University Press, 1985). Morantz-Sanchez demonstrates that nineteenth-century female physicians incorporated yet transcended traditional domestic ideology. For infant feeding, see Rima D. Apple, *Mothers and Medicine: A Social History of Infant Feeding, 1890–1950* (Madison: University of Wisconsin Press, 1987); Judith Walzer Leavitt, *Brought to Bed; Childbearing in America, 1750–1950* (New York: Oxford University Press); Richard A. Meckel, *Save the Babies: American Public Health Reform and the Prevention of Infant Mortality, 1850–1929* (Baltimore: The Johns Hopkins University Press, 1990).

11. Kathleen Jones, "Sentiment and Science: The Late Nineteenth Century Pediatrician as Mother's Advisor," *Journal of Social History* 17 (1983): 84–85; Halpern, *American Pediatrics*, 84–85.

12. Stephen J. Leonard and Thomas J. Noel, *Denver: From Mining Camp to Metropolis* (Niwot: University Press of Colorado, 1990), 16–17, 91, 110.

13. Typescript, "George Byron Packard, Sr., MD," n.d., typescript in Children's Hospital of Denver Collection (hereinafter referred to as CHD Collection).

14. "G. Robert Fisher, M.D., 1916–1924," n.d., typescript included in series of physician profiles in CHD Collection (hereinafter referred to as Physician Profiles). Additional sources consulted for biographical information include the annual reports of The Children's Hospital; Colorado Medical Society *Century of Colorado Medicine, Jubilee Volume*; and the CHD Collection.

15. Ibid.

16. Shikes, *Rocky Mountain Medicine*, 94–95.

17. "Dr. Minnie Love Dies Following 10-Day Illness," *Denver Post*, May 13, 1942; *Rocky Mountain News*, May 13, 1942; typescript, "Mrs. Charles Gurley Love (Dr. Minnie C.T. Love)," #46139 in CHD Collection; Shikes, *Rocky Mountain Medicine*, 97, reports Charles R. Love's death from tuberculosis. Shikes's sources for information on Dr. Love include: M. De Mund, *Women Physicians of Colorado* (Denver, 1976), 64; Mary Reed Stratton, M.D., manuscript compilation of biographies of Colorado's women physicians, Denver Medical Society Library; M.C.T. Love, "Women Practitioners of Colorado," Transactions of the Colorado State Medical Society 32:503, 1901.

18. Oca Cushman's maiden name was probably Rush, as her brother was John W. Rush from Holden. She had two sisters, named Mary Jane Rice of Tulsa, Oklahoma, and Gertrude Thompson of Pasadena, California. Untitled manuscript, n.d., CHD Collection.

19. Janet C. Cunningham, R.N., m.s., "Early Nursing, The Children's Hospital, Denver, Colorado; The First Decade, 1910–1920," n.d., typescript provided to the author. Cunningham used some of the following sources for her paper: Nolie Mumey, *Cap, Pin and Diploma; A History of the Colorado Training School, the Oldest in the State for Nurses* (Boulder: Johnson Publishing Co., 1968); Lillian DeYoung, "The Genesis of Saint Luke's Hospital School of Nursing," typescript in the Denver Presbyterian/St. Luke's Hospital School of Nursing Archive Collection (hereinafter cited as SLH Archives), Denver; Louie Croft Boyd, Scrap-

book of Nursing Legislation in Colorado, 1905-1946, typescript; St. Luke's Hospital Bulletin, Chapter 11, 1893, "The Philosophy, Aims, Objectives of Curriculum; Constitution, By-laws, and Rules," SLH Archives; Janet Cunningham interview with Dr. C. Richard Hawes, retired cardiologist, October 11, 1990; Cunningham interview with Alice Alcott, R.N., retired, November 3, 1987; and Winifred Moss interview with Alcott, October 9, 1990.

20. Leonard and Noel, *Mining Camp to Metropolis*, 91–100.

21. Claire McCausland, *An Element of Love: A History of the Children's Memorial Hospital of Chicago, Illinois* (Chicago: The Children's Memorial Hospital, 1981), 31–32; Clement A. Smith, *The Children's Hospital of Boston: "Built Better Than They Knew"* (Boston and Toronto: Little, Brown and Co., 1983), 113–114.

22. *Rocky Mountain News*, June 19, 1897.

23. Seymour E. Wheelock, M.D., "Three Centuries in an Hour; An Overview of the History of Child Care in Colorado." Paper presented to the Gengenbach Society in Denver, Spring 1983, 16–20.

24. Ibid., 20.

25. *Denver Post*, May 13, 1942.

Chapter 2

A Hospital Is Born

Despite numerous public causes competing for their attention at the turn of the century, prominent Denver women remained aware of the needs of the region's disadvantaged children. Supported by male and female colleagues, Dr. Love once again initiated a project to care for the city's sick children. A meeting of Denver club women was held on April 5, 1906, at 978 Logan Street, the home of Mrs. Hattie C. Colburn. Dr. Love emphasized the great need in Denver for a special hospital for sick and crippled children; she was supported by two other female physicians, Eleanor Lawney and Ethel V. Fraser. Four of the women drafted constitution and bylaws. They named the prospective facility the Blanche Roosevelt Hospital, after Dr. Love's sister who had married into the Roosevelt family; the women clearly sought her financial support. In fact, Dr. Love donated the first $100, pledging $500 more in the first year. Three other women gave $100 each, another $50, and several others pledged $5 per year.

Later that year Dr. Love articulated the association's goals at length, the challenges facing "many well-known Denver ladies noted for their broad and efficient work among the poor and needy of the city." She continued:

> The cause of sick crippled children needs no advocate. . . . As soon as sufficient money and furnishings are pledged . . . a suitable house will be procured and fitted out with all the modern appliances for the successful treatment of the acute and chronic diseases of children. . . . In a hospital devoted exclusively to children the little patients are free from subjection to sights and sounds not best for them to see and hear, but which are unavoidable among the adult sick.[1]

Dr. Love had hoped the Roosevelt name would stimulate the generosity of the local elite. But President Theodore Roosevelt was disliked among erstwhile western Populists. Silver miners were still recovering from the federal adherence to the gold standard, a large factor in the Depression of 1893 from which Colorado still suffered. Moreover his

federal land and conservation policies were controversial among agricul-
tural, cattle, and lumber interests. The Rockefeller medical philanthropies
were prestigious in the East; the West was different. Nevertheless two
national politicians responded to the newly named institution: Thomas
Patterson gave $1,000, and future senator Lawrence Phipps donated
$5,000.[2]

At a second meeting, female incorporators were nominated and
approved. The Blanche Roosevelt Association was incorporated on May 6,
1906. Bylaws included provisions for recognition of charitable donations
and guaranteed female control of the association, which was typical of
children's hospitals in the nation. Life memberships in The Blanche
Roosevelt Hospital for Children Association were $100; a one-year free bed
in the donor's name was $250.[3]

The women did not anticipate inflation that would render these
amounts insufficient for maintaining even a single hospital bed. Several
years later "undervaluing" hospital rooms and beds remained a problem
for the female directors at Children's Hospital. In late 1912 the female
president of Mercy Hospital, a facility for children in Kansas City, Missouri,
offered friendly criticism of fund-raising strategies documented in The
Children's Hospital annual report. She pointed out her own institution's
flawed fund-raising techniques:

> We named a number of rooms in perpetuity. The ones for whom they were
> named paid us from $150 to $800 for this privilege. This money was supposed
> to pay for the actual building of the room and . . . was not nearly sufficient
> for the building or the upkeeping of it. We have forever handicapped our-
> selves, because human nature is a good deal alike all over the world, and one
> person is not apt to desire to do anything for a room named in honor of
> someone else.

She cautioned against awarding life memberships too cheaply: "We also
have a life membership of $100. We regret it, because life members are
usually people of means, and this $100 in a measure debars us from further
solicitation."[4]

One organizing principle of the hospital for children suggested acceptance of a widely held view that women were in their proper domestic
sphere in overseeing the care of sick children. The board of directors
excluded men for fully six decades, until December 1968. Like their outspo-

ken eastern sisters Denver club women did not abide by strict social convention; they used their own rather than their husbands' names.[5]

Professional women also clearly voiced a desire for authority. The bylaws asserted that "at least one half of the medical officers shall be women physicians." Other sections reinforced strict professionalism and the highest educational standards in a new era of hospitals founded upon modern administration and increasingly strict medical profession standards. Bylaws suggested that the Denver venture would be somewhat more scientifically oriented than the New York and Chicago hospitals for children. This may simply have reflected the fact that by the later date of its incorporation, the medical profession as a whole had far more scientific authority. Yet the hospital's community and humanitarian purposes remained constant. The female founders successfully bridged the transition of U.S. hospitals for children from charitable to predominantly scientific institutions.

Some legal shuffling was necessary in the early years. The women directors reincorporated on May 2, 1907, changed the name to The Children's Hospital Association, reincorporated yet again on May 9, 1908, and appointed four men advisors.[6] A handful of directors dropped out, and new ones were elected. Dr. Love's direct involvement ceased. On August 13, 1908, the board reported the purchase of nine lots at Albion and Sixteenth Avenue for $1,200. On September 10, $3,177.26 was reported in the treasury.[7]

Over the next few months association leaders quietly attracted contributions and other forms of support. The building fund in particular gained critical support of prominent Denverites. In November 1908 dramatic events began to unfold. Mrs. Frederick G. Bonfils reported that the *Denver Post* wanted to support hospital construction in the amount of $4,000–$5,000 in Christmas party proceeds. She hoped that two spring "entertainments" would net another $10,000.[8] But there was bad news as well. The association was startled to learn that their treasurer, Electra Beard, had managed either to lose or abscond with the treasury.[9]

After Christmas the executive committee firmly confronted the significant embarrassment to their benevolent endeavor. Mrs. Beard admitted embezzling $2,119.60. The board's minutes stated: "She still refused to give the name or names of parties interested with her in the transaction, but was willing to give her whole life to the making of restitution to the Association." She surrendered the deed to her heavily mortgaged house at 1545 Steele Street and its contents and furniture.

In a meeting on January 14, 1909, ladies of the board resolved but then tabled an impassioned resolution condemning Mrs. Beard for "commission of such crimes [which] are among the most flagrant, contemptible and unpardonable" and urged prosecution to the full extent of the law. The club women declared her an outcast. The resolution continued: "If by reason of judicial clemency she should retain her freedom, all clubs, societies, and institutions be warned against the said Mrs. Beard, as unworthy of trust or confidence."[10]

The police arrested her. She admitted that she had "just simply spent" the money. Further, even after her theft was discovered, she had continued to solicit funds as if still representing the association. Mrs. Beard was released when the association agreed not to press charges if she made restitution. Unfortunately this action did not contain the damage to the association's reputation, and the incident was divisive. Electra Beard was a working woman, but she freely volunteered her time, perhaps thereby clinging to middle-class status. In addition to her work with the association, she was historian for the Daughters of the American Revolution and was a Colonial Dame. Yet she had a checkered past. She had lost her job as marriage clerk at the courthouse because she had sent applicants to a "well-known Methodist minister" and received kickbacks of $8 to $10 per month from him. Even for petty graft, the amount was small.[11]

The board affirmed the association's integrity and continued with its social mission. Although the Beard incident was unfortunate — the final loss was $1,247[12] — it only delayed but did not prevent opening a hospital for children. In the meantime, the directors and other volunteers overcame the obstacle and raised funds by traditional means. A bazaar netted at least $1,146 from sale of fifty-seven dolls, 135 "candies," and eighty-four "fancy articles"; $1,500 was netted at another doll bazaar; a picnic at Elitch's raised $2,933; $1,305 came from a charity ball. The association received twenty-five cents a ticket from the Shriner's Circus and $163 from another fair. Finally, on August 11, 1909, the directors recorded purchase of a house with 3.5 lots at 2221 Downing Street, for $15,729.[13]

The house, once owned by Dr. Horace G. Wetherill, was formally dedicated as the Denver Maternity and Woman's Hospital in 1902 and boasted eighteen beds, two of which were endowed. The association perceived a need to remodel the building.[14] At first they called it a "boarding

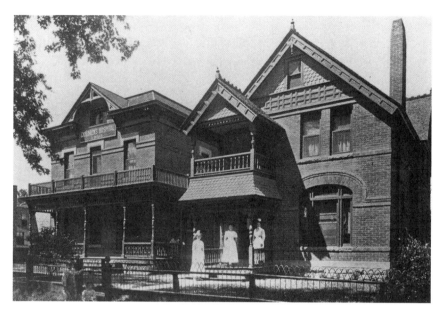

First site for the hospital and nurses' training school located at 2221 Downing Street.

house," perhaps to prevent neighborhood residents from opposing the location and possible expansion of a full-fledged hospital there. The association had already encountered neighborhood opposition elsewhere; the board had not developed the nine lots at Albion and Sixteenth because it had failed to gain neighborhood consent, which by law was two-thirds of property owners. Downing Street neighbors were also wary. "The property owners allege," the Denver *Times* reported on December 12, 1909, "that their holdings will be materially decreased in value, that the hospital will spread disease among them and cause illness in their families and otherwise endanger them."[15]

Mrs. E. W. Williams, president of the board, made an impassioned response to the neighborhood injunction, which hung "like a thunder cloud over . . . the association." She asserted: "A charity of this kind is so badly needed in Denver, and the majority of people living near the building have assured us that they are in sympathy with the movement." She concluded

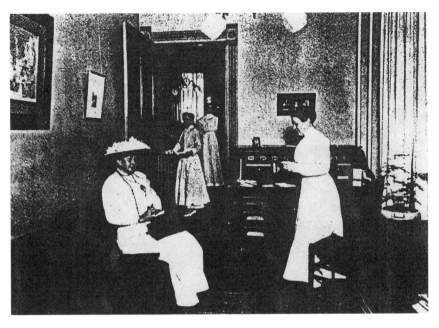

Office located at 2221 Downing; Oca Cushman is standing at desk.

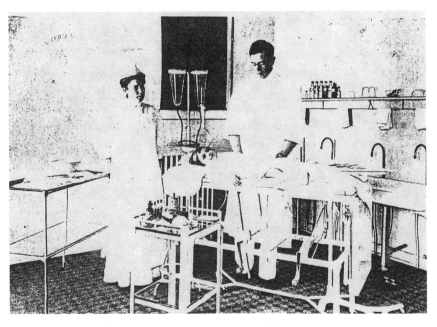

Partial view of operating room at 2221 Downing.

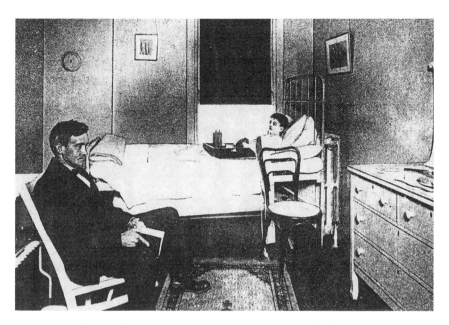

"James Robert Burger Room," a private room in the first hospital.

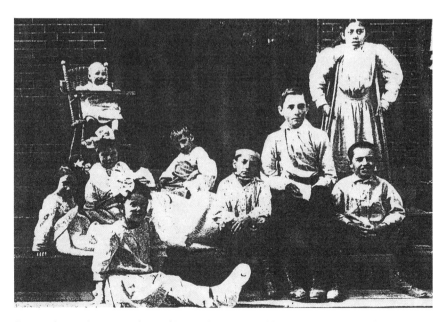

Group of convalescents in front of hospital. Ten-year-old Constantia Esquibel from Rincon, New Mexico (top right), was admitted with serious neuromuscular complications from a neglected case of infantile paralysis. After two years in the hospital she was able to walk unsupported.

that "if it were not for old-time friendships they would have signed our petition."[16] Mrs. Williams lamented a general opposition to institutions for the underprivileged in prosperous neighborhoods. According to two prominent Denver historians, the Ladies' Relief Society asylum for homeless children established at 800 Logan in 1876 had been demolished in 1897 "to relieve the affluent Capitol Hill neighborhood of 'unsightliness.' "[17] The Downing Street house was a lying-in hospital, a function perhaps more acceptable to local residents than that of the new institution, which would serve diseased children, some poor and minority. Mrs. Williams tried to reassure neighbors: "The hospital is not a home in any sense of the word, the children will be seen very rarely in the yard, for when a child is well enough to play in the yard it will be sent home, and when it is sick enough to stay at the hospital it will be kept indoors, except as it may be placed in a lawn chair to get the benefit of the open air and sunshine."[18] Yet she also spoke of a "fight" and aggressive efforts to "bitterly combat" neighborhood opponents. The women were determined not to lose the approximately $3,000 already spent on remodeling in preparation for an expected opening by January 1, 1910.[19] One remark proved to be highly ironic. Mrs. Williams concluded: "When it is completed we will have room for from twenty to thirty children, but I do not suppose that we will be full more than half the time."[20]

Young patients were considered as individuals, a symbol of their special status in the West but also reflecting a holistic view of the child as part of the larger community. The press touted the hospital's homey setting. One article repeated the idyllic portrait of the 1897 tent encampment: a sun-lit atmosphere, with healthy-looking children in crisp white surroundings and nursery figures gaily adorning the walls. Oca Cushman, destined to play a major role in running The Children's Hospital for the next forty-five years, was dubbed "the genial mother."[21]

Nursing was a profession for young women willing to live cloistered lives of dedication to patient care. The hospital was the nurse's home, the patients and staff her family. Oca Cushman had worked for seven years at nearby St. Luke's and had served as night supervisor. While at St. Luke's, she had tended the husband of Mrs. C. H. Abbott, a board member at Children's. He was so impressed that he recommended Mrs. Cushman for a job at Children's. Thus was Oca Cushman appointed superintendent at Children's Hospital when it opened on February 17, 1910. The director of nurses was Miss Marguerite Bullene.[22] Mrs. Cushman took care of admis-

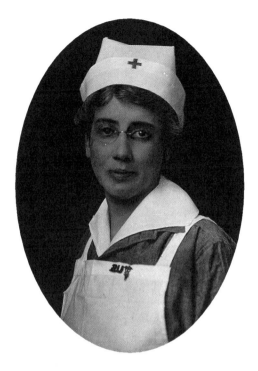

Miss Marguerite Bullene, R.N., superintendent of
the Training School for Nurses.

sions, attended daily rounds with the physicians, did all the hiring and
firing, and maintained the good order and sanitation at the Downing Street
house.

Recollections of Mrs. Cushman's long tenure are vivid. She "literally
worked her way through the halls wearing white gloves, fingering ledges
for dust." She exercised her prerogative as matriarch in the care of Denver's
children, even over federal authorities. She moved the mailbox to a location
she thought preferable to the one chosen by the U.S. Post Office, and postal
authorities let it remain. Mrs. Cushman seemingly handled just about
everything. She was head seamstress, sewing nurses' uniforms and adding
frills to patients' Christmas frocks. She controlled the daily diet, conducting
this chore with a touch of the farmer's wife by making jams, jellies, soups,
and pies. Her patients received good-night kisses until one of them gave
her measles. She also acted as grande dame over the mostly male medical

staff. Like the female directors, she raised funds, in particular attracting the attention of the Tammens.[23]

By the time it closed in 1956, the Training School for Nurses had graduated 502 women. Thousands of other affiliated students also received training at this school. Hospital records outlined precise social, moral, and intellectual standards. Acceptance required at least one year of high school or the equivalent; the commitment included two years of training to deal with diseases in children under sixteen. Courses entailed lectures from physicians, surgeons, and the superintendent of nurses, as well as four months' off-campus general duty in an adult ward and two months in obstetrical training. Trainees studied anatomy, physiology, hygiene, materia medica, infant feeding, medical and surgical diseases of children, bacteriology, prophylaxis, gynecology, and dietetics. Students had a two-month probationary period but could be dismissed at any time.

Their education was nearly complete compensation for exacting services. In addition to board, lodging, and laundry, trainees received $6 a month the first year, $8 the second, and $10 per month the last six months. This was "to defray the cost of uniforms, text books and expenses incidental to training, and not . . . personal necessities." Shifts lasted twelve hours, changing at 7:30 A.M. and 7:30 P.M. Day nurses were allowed two hours off duty a day, one afternoon each week, and half of Sunday.

Standards of personal hygiene and behavior were precise. Age limits for applicants were eighteen to thirty years. Moreover, they had to be "strong and healthy, able to read aloud well and take notes at lectures. . . . The teeth must be in good condition . . . and applicants must show satisfactory evidence of recent vaccination." Dress was carefully prescribed; complete conformity was expected, especially during the two-month probation period.

> During probation pupils will need three plain gingham dresses; ten white aprons made of 10-quarter sheeting, with hem six inches wide, to reach to the bottom of the skirt, a one-inch hem down the back, a band two inches wide fastened at the back with two buttons; one wrapper; a full supply of underclothing, plainly marked; two laundry bags; shoes with rubber heels; a pair of surgical scissors and a napkin ring. Every article to be marked with owner's name in full. A watch with a second hand, and a thermometer will also be needed. Candidates coming from a distance must provide themselves with money for their return traveling expenses in case they are not accepted as pupil-nurses.[24]

Subsequent reports for 1910 indicated problems with such exacting standards and so rigid a personal code. Superintendent Bullene wrote that the number of applicants was "discouragingly small, other schools having experienced the same difficulty." Fourteen applications had been accepted, but at year's end she reported only six current pupils and three probationers.[25]

Attrition declined the following year. Eleven nurses and probationers were active, with two more on duty at St. Joseph's. Four nurses came from the Fort Collins Training School for three months, plus one pupil from the Fort Collins Hospital. Miss Bullene emphasized the educational advantages of additional training at other nearby hospitals. The Children's medical and surgical staff also gave numerous lectures. In 1911 the curriculum was lengthened from two and a half to three years to enhance preparation for the state board examination.[26]

Images of charity and childhood innocence permeated early annual reports, which conveyed many gems of traditional Victorian morality but even stronger strains of individualism, voluntarism, and egalitarianism. The *First Annual Report* included an exact ethnic profile of patients. Of the 291 patients, 212 were born in the United States. There were thirty-three Hebrew, ten each Italian and German, four Swedish, and three or fewer from thirteen other countries. The account covered only from February 17 to April 1, 1910.[27]

Children with contagious diseases were sent to Steele Hospital, located at Cherokee and West Seventh Avenue, the city's contagious facility; in addition, children with "chronic" or "incurable" illness or disease were not admitted unless treatment would relieve symptoms. Thus mortality remained low, avoiding a depressing environment that was unappealing to the majority of paying parents who eventually helped make the hospital financially successful.[28]

In 1912 a visiting committee chaired by Ena Stahl expanded the hospital's mission to include visits of charity patients. Mrs. Stahl envisioned home aftercare as a permanent part of the visiting committee's "uplift work." But the women established clear limits on charity work. Although about a third of the children treated the first year received full or part payment as charity, only one-sixth or forty-seven children were fully supported by association benevolence.[29] In 1912 the amount spent on charity patients more than doubled, but paying patients contributed over

$7,500 to the hospital's receipts. The mortality rate remained low at only sixteen out of 348 patients.[30]

Reflecting the increasing appeal of hospital care because of more effective surgery and therapeutics, the women directors offered free beds "to those who are really poor," but all others would pay "a moderate charge." At first there were only two free beds: one endowed by the Lawrence C. Phipps family, the other by the proceeds of the "Good Samaritan" bazaar. Both beds were first filled by crippled little girls. A five-year-old girl with hip disease was brought from Delta County, then "relieved from pain by proper appliances." The second bed was filled by a small Mexican girl from Rincon, New Mexico, named Constantia, who had never walked, having contracted polio as an infant.[31] She became the star of the fledgling public relations efforts at Denver's new private, voluntary hospital for children.

Constantia entered the new hospital in April 1910. Dr. George B. Packard, Sr., performed successful surgery. Four months later Constantia appeared with crutches, wearing a brace but moving about freely. The *Denver Post,* through a special human relations fund, promised to maintain her at the hospital for a year or longer. "Surely," the paper proclaimed, "subscribers who supported the endeavor must feel a thrill of exhilaration. Moreover, the managers of the Hospital feel that the benefit derived by this one child is more than a sufficient justification for the hospital's existence!"[32]

After less than a year of operation, Dr. Love, although no longer associated directly with the hospital, offered praise to the founders: "The management is to be congratulated in every particular: the generosity of its patrons in providing three free beds for the children of the poor, the beautiful and thoroughly scientific equipment, and the splendid medical and surgical staff. May it grow and prosper and prove to be a source of new life and health to thousands of little ones."[33] Though charity cases tugged at donors' heartstrings, dramatic healing enhanced the appeal among the affluent of a medical institution for children. New curative and public health efforts began to alleviate some crippling diseases such as bovine tuberculosis. Long-term treatment with special equipment and appliances promised vast improvement in children's lives.

The female directors maintained a steady vigil over the needy sick children of Denver. While persistently emphasizing the nonsectarian nature of Children's Hospital, board president Mrs. Williams made it clear

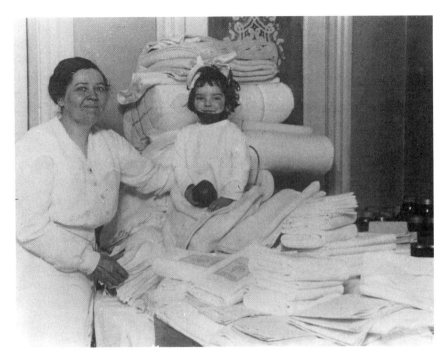

Sample of the proceeds from the 1915 Donation Day; these were later transformed by volunteers at sewing bees into linens, nightgowns, and other useful items.

that gifts were a continuing part of a Christian stewardship: "The charity which this institution represents appeals to the tenderest and broadest Christian philanthropy, for the hospital is peculiarly a Christian institution." Doctors and board members gave freely of furnishings, equipment, and a plethora of "miscellaneous donations" creating a homelike atmosphere. Gifts included jellies, fruit, potatoes, flowers, pillows, sheets, blankets, toys, clothes, baskets, chickens, and even rabbits for Easter. Every donor and donation was listed in early reports.[34]

Community physicians could also refer patients to the hospital with the assurance they would "receive every attention." Superintendent Cushman controlled admissions, but accident cases were not screened. The board touted "liberal" visiting hours from 2:00 to 4:00 P.M.[35] The women emphasized the balance maintained between "housekeeping" and "technical" efficiency and keeping a cheerful atmosphere in describing Superintendent Cushman's domain: "The superintendent aims to have her house in good order every afternoon, not especial order on certain days. Children's toys and snips of cutting paper lying about in the wards are not disorder, but tokens of happiness. Every afternoon at half past four these are put away and the floors swept." The medical staff was reportedly "well pleased" with the material environment; they also found the surroundings attractive for their paying patients.[36] The founders of Children's Hospital articulated a clear, future objective that still prevails eighty years later: "We hope to become well-known enough, and large enough, to take care of all the children; but we also hope that we may never become so large that we have cases instead of individuals — numbers instead of names."[37]

The structure of the medical and surgical staff indicated the growing complexity and specialization of the profession. Perhaps because of the paucity of female physicians, the organizers could not honor the original bylaw that half the medical executive committee be female. The first female member was Laura L. Liebhardt, M.D., followed by Dr. Eleanor Lawney.[38] Notable additions to the medical and surgical staff were Drs. George B. Packard, Sr., Leonard W. Ely, and H. W. Wilcox.[39] All of these doctors, male and female, had joined the staff by the end of 1911.

Because no children with contagious diseases were admitted to Children's, tonsil and adenoid surgery ("T&As") was one of the principal procedures performed at the hospital.[40] The anesthesia staff also grew from one visiting physician to three between 1915 and 1920.[41] Ophthalmology and otology expanded under Drs. Melville Black, Edgar F. Conant, and Elmer E. McKeown. Minnie Love's son, T. R. Love, joined Henry S. Denison in pathology. Dr. Love later became secretary of the State Board of Health, following his mother's career path in public health.[42]

Other additions to the hospital "family" were eight nurses under Superintendent Bullene, and a thirty-one-member men's advisory board, including such prominent figures as board chairman C. B. Kountze, James Brown, Walter Cheesman, Rodney Curtis, and William G. Evans.[43] Dual commitments by both spouses in some families, among the women's board of directors, the men's advisory board, and the medical and surgical staff, were common. Running Children's Hospital was often a family affair.

By the end of the first year the treasurer noted that the "average number of patients has steadily increased from twelve to the full capacity of thirty, and four or five extra beds have been crowded in to accommodate . . . those seeking the benefits of the Hospital." Incredibly, the daily average cost per patient was $1.46. A total of $1,967.27 was expended for charity.

One hundred and sixty operations had been performed.[44] Hip-joint disease was the most common orthopaedic condition: twenty-three boys and ten girls were afflicted. T&As combined for fifty-five cases. Another orthopaedic condition, clubfoot, accounted for fifteen cases, twelve male and three female. Clubfoot corrections were apparently a highly successful endeavor and drew the largest percentage of patients from outside the city. They also were treated aggressively as "bloodless operations" and had a 100 percent improvement and discharge rate.[45]

Skeletal tuberculosis dominated the large orthopaedic caseload. This situation was typical for children's hospitals nationwide because of the bovine strain of the tubercle bacillus in unsterilized and unpasteurized milk. At Boston Children's Hospital central features of its patient profile from 1882 to 1914 were large increases in orthopaedic and surgical tuberculosis cases. But even in the rarified intellectual environment of Boston, doctors did not yet recognize the impact of infected milk on children's health.

At Denver Children's Hospital, tubercular orthopaedic cases and congenital deformities accounted for 104 manipulation and cast cases in 1912, surpassed only by 106 T&As. The T&As continued to rise, while orthopaedic cases remained stationary, greatly declining in relative importance during the hospital's first decades.[46] According to one doctor-historian at Children's Hospital, T&A surgery was "up for grabs" among new pediatric specialists and general practitioners. By the 1930s the surgery would become a boon for struggling pediatricians attempting to make ends meet; it was performed on poor children for as little as $15, divided equally among the hospital, the anesthetist, and the surgeon.[47]

A new disease appeared in children's orthopaedic wards. During 1911 one case of infantile paralysis and three of "neglected poliomyelitis" were admitted; one child died.[48] The following year the figures were seven and one. Similarly, medical and surgical staff tasks showed subtle but significant changes as "Infant Feeding" was separated from "General Medicine." Drs. J. W. Amesse, F. P. Gengenbach, and H. B. Whitney proclaimed themselves pediatric specialists and endorsed the national public health movement to "save the babies" from the ravages of contaminated milk and infant diarrhea.[49] Simultaneously, the primacy of orthopaedic surgery declined with the vast improvement in urban milk supplies and implementation of state sanitation and pasteurization laws.

Specialization also marked the organizational evolution of the hospital's board of directors. The first board had four standing committees: building, house, finance, and membership. The annual report for 1912 listed several new committees: work, training school, kindergarten, monthly visitors, and a "clinic committee." The participation of many prominent Denver businessmen on the Investment and Advisory Committee testified to the commitment of Denver's social and economic leaders.[50]

Mrs. George B. Packard, Sr., served on the board for twenty-four years. Her early history of the hospital, published in 1934, combined affectionate sentimentality for Denver's sick children with a pragmatic account of nuts-and-bolts building and fund-raising during the program's first quarter-century. She also chaired the Membership Committee, which raised funds for charity patients. Personal gifts supporting work accomplished at 2221 Downing dominated early contributions. The needs met by the women were within their abilities as homemakers, wives, and mothers — largely food, clothing, and toys. Although the dollar amounts appear inconceivable in the late twentieth century, this generosity and other efficiencies lowered the original cost per patient from $1.46 a day to $1.18 in 1912.[51]

The Packard family symbolized the integration of family and professional life among early Children's Hospital supporters. Dr. George Packard, Sr., a surgeon, was appointed professor of orthopaedics when the University of Colorado Medical School was established in Denver in 1892. Elected president of the American Orthopaedic Association in 1914, he was renowned for research and treatment of childhood bone tuberculosis and congenital deformities.[52]

Both Packard sons established careers in Denver. Robert G. Packard graduated from Northwestern University with an M.D. degree in 1912, then returned to Denver and worked with his father until World War I, when he served in Europe. Robert Packard became interested in orthopaedic treatment of fractures, and after his return to Denver in 1919, he abandoned conservative methods of manipulations, casts, and braces, favoring open surgery in bone and joint tuberculosis and congenital deformities (dislocated hips, clubfoot).[53]

George B. Packard, Jr., graduated from the University of Colorado and Harvard University School of Medicine. He completed surgical training at Massachusetts General Hospital and returned to Colorado about 1921. He performed the first Ramstedt operation in Denver. This procedure involved incising and thereby loosening a muscle located at the outlet of an infant's stomach, permitting food to pass through. When overly tight and constricted, the muscle causes pyloric stenosis, characterized by unremitting vomiting. Dr. Packard was less specialized in orthopaedic surgery than his father and brother and remained a general pediatric surgeon.[54] He was instrumental in further improving pediatric surgery at the end of World War II. While head of the Department of Surgery at the University of Colorado Medical School, he helped Children's Hospital qualify for accreditation in its residency training program. In 1945–1946, he also initiated the Infant Surgery Ward and helped add an intensive care unit and other surgical facilities.[55]

The Packard name and the benefits from the family's perceptive devotion to the often-convoluted affairs of The Children's Hospital did not disappear with the death of Dr. George Packard, Jr. His daughter, Carol Packard Tempest, was a forthright member of the board of directors during many critical hours, supplementing her intramural energies with the insights gained as an elected state representative and as a lobbyist for the Colorado Medical Society in the state legislature.

Still, the early regional physicians in orthopaedic surgery often seemed to personify what English socialist and medical reformer Beatrice Webb found in her 1898 visit to Denver. She claimed that Denverites had "a restless admiration for Eastern America, an uneasy consciousness of their inferiority to New York, Boston or Philadelphia, a dread of the ridicule of the Eastern newspapers, a desire that their children should have the advantages of an 'Eastern' education."[56]

Eastern-born physicians came to Denver along with tens of thousands of other health seekers. Henry W. Wilcox trained and worked with Dr. Packard, Sr., beginning in 1902. Like his mentor he came west because of pulmonary tuberculosis. He graduated from the University of Colorado Medical School in 1897. A colleague described him as "the good shepherd of the crippled," saying that his nonpecuniary attitude made many poorer people gravitate to him. Wilcox remained active on the Children's Hospital staff until his retirement in 1947.[57]

S. Fosdick Jones received his undergraduate degree from Massachusetts Institute of Technology and his M.D. from Columbia University College of Physicians. He went first to Pasadena to recover from poor health, then began practice in Denver in 1906. After 1914 he assisted Dr. Packard at the University of Colorado, entered military service in 1917, and returned in 1919. He was appointed chief of the Orthopaedic Department at the university in 1924, holding the position until 1928, when poor health forced him into early retirement.[58]

Many eastern-trained doctors established a pattern that has persisted to the present, dividing their time between the university and Children's Hospital. Demand for treatment at the latter quickly tested the managerial abilities of volunteer directors. The annual report for 1911 noted that the hospital had been running at full capacity. The average stay was 24.5 days; some spent an entire year strapped to frames to correct orthopaedic conditions. "Physicians have urged us to enlarge the Hospital," Clara Williams declared, "and this should be done as soon as possible."

Along with domestic comfort, the imperatives of science and technology were important to the volunteers. Mrs. Williams recommended addition of an outpatient department, a "room and apparatus for X-ray and other electrical work," plus a large room equipped with "appliances for instruction and practice in Swedish movements and corrective gymnastics" for orthopaedic cases. The hospital needed a contagion ward for "suspicious cases" and an "isolation building."[59]

Clearly the converted dwelling at 2221 Downing Street would not suffice for long. In the summer of 1911 the *Rocky Mountain News* reported that hospital management was planning "a large, well-equipped and strictly modern and thoroughly up-to-date hospital for these little sufferers." Every child deserved the "chance to recover their birthright, a strong healthy physical body." The paper claimed that despite the crowded conditions, scientific standards were uncompromising: "The staff of the hospital is composed largely of specialists in children's diseases. The hospital itself is a model of cleanliness, and the service at the highest standard."[60]

At 2221 Downing Street space was planned for thirty children, but forty-four could be crowded in. In 1909 the association had purchased twelve lots at Nineteenth and Downing, partly from the $8,000 treasury of the County Hospital Children's Pavilion, which consolidated with Children's. The lots cost $12,011, and the treasury had $10,000 more for a building fund. During 1912–1913 admissions doubled, and a new building became a critical priority. The April 3, 1914, board minutes once again focused on "woeful lack of space" at the old facility, resulting in "almost daily refusals to both physicians and patients."[61]

Despite the distractions of World War I, Denver's assertive female philanthropists forged ahead with plans for a new hospital. Perhaps fol-

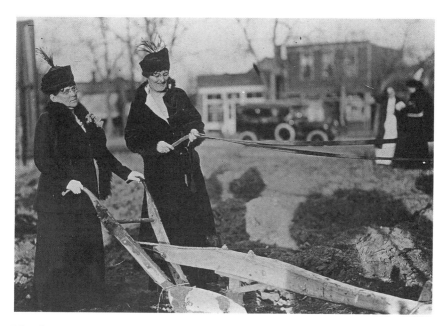

Mrs. George B. Packard, Sr., second vice president, and Mrs. James C. Burger, president, breaking ground for the new Children's Hospital, Nineteenth Avenue at Downing Street, February 14, 1916.

lowing the advice of eastern-trained physicians, the women eschewed local architects. They chose the firm of Biscoe and Morman of Boston, with Dr. S. S. Goldwater of New York as a consultant. Frederick C. Barber of New York directed a $250,000 building campaign. Fifty volunteer teams convened for a dinner at the Albany Hotel. Fortified with inspiration as well as victuals, they raised over $211,000 in ten days! The estimated building cost was $182,000 (the actual cost was $194,000).[62] Ground breaking occurred on February 24, 1916, attended by an audience estimated from 500 to "thousands." The board hired Merritt Gano, Sr., to supervise construction; financier Harold Kountze, whose wife was active on the board, distributed all funds.[63]

The new Children's Hospital opened on February 12, 1917. Typically the *Denver Post* painted an idyllic, sentimental scene. The nurses at the old Downing Street house "began their work of bathing and dressing every mite in their care and getting ready wraps that were to keep them from taking cold on their ride to the new building." Nurses and doctors took the

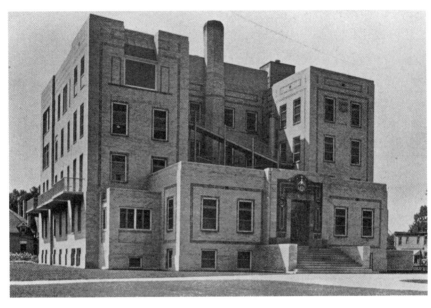

The new Children's Hospital located at Nineteenth Avenue at Downing Street.

thirty "little bundles of humanity in their arms" from their beds at 2221 Downing to the new hospital building.[64]

The new building was a technological marvel, facilitating more complex and expanded care. Efficiencies included electric elevators, a modern fire escape, porches, and balconies. Every ward had sterilizing equipment, a kitchen with refrigeration, steam tables and gas for cooking, special bathing areas for patients, modern plumbing, closets, and steam blanket warmers. Each floor also had a laundry chute and a dumbwaiter from the main kitchen.[65] An isolation ward was a concession to the reality of contagious urban disease in the 1910s, and the needs of poor and working-class children. Middle- and upper-class children with contagious diseases were usually treated at home, often under quarantine, with house calls by private practitioners, some of whom also practiced at Children's Hospital.

In 1916 there was an unprecedented polio epidemic on the East Coast. It had little immediate regional impact in Denver, where Children's reported only nine cases. All were treated as orthopaedic cases; only one was cured, but seven "improved." The annual report for 1918 noted only six polio cases. By contrast there were forty-three orthopaedic cases, twenty-six clubfoot corrections, and twenty-three scoliosis cases. Seventy-five children with cleft palate and harelips all were reported cured. Other medical and surgical cases in 1918 included thirty appendectomies, ninety-five infant feeding cases, and seventy-eight T&As.[66] Subsequent reports reflected the growing complexity of pediatrics, with cases listed by organ systems, diseases, and procedures.[67]

In 1915 and 1916 the hospital's patients were mostly paying, with only 13.7 percent receiving complete or partial charity. The mortality rate remained low with sixty-nine deaths, about 3 percent. Administrators screened charity cases carefully in order not to overextend limited reserves. Services did not extend to contagious diseases, those deemed incurable or chronic, unless they could be significantly "relieved" by hospital treatment.[68] Hospital leaders prized an optimistic, cheery atmosphere, avoiding the old stereotype of urban hospitals as asylums for poor, dying, and destitute children.

In 1920 board president Mabel G. Hodges carefully delineated the boundary between private and public responsibility, charting the voluntary nonsectarian yet philanthropic mission of the Children's Hospital Association. "The County Hospital is maintained by the people for charity service, and our function should be . . . to render that service when the County Hospital is unable to do it or in those instances where our members, having special interest in some individual case, desire the service." She warned that to "solicit charity work or attempt to divert it from the County Hospital" would overwhelm their resources. Yet constant expansion of charity work was necessitated by the expanding needs of the city. She called for larger endowments to enable continuing increase in charity service, "that field which brings us the most gratifying sense of accomplishment."[69]

By nurturing ideals of science and efficiency instead of a house of refuge for the hopeless, Children's leaders enhanced community support for their endeavor. Nevertheless, contagion was a continual fear because of physical crowding and charity cases admitted without accurate health reports. Children with "suspicious symptoms" were promptly discharged after "rigid daily inspections." The hospital forged a temporary agreement whereby the city health department removed patients if epidemic disease appeared among patients held for two weeks in two small isolation wards. This unsatisfactory arrangement was soon abandoned in favor of a separate house converted to an isolation unit accommodating ten or twelve patients. This separate facility was expensive, however, and the staff continually feared cross-infection.[70]

In the waning months of World War I another crisis evolved, in the form of an international influenza epidemic claiming millions of victims. Between September 1918 and June 1919 the epidemic killed more than 1,500 Denverites, one out of nine of the 13,000 afflicted in the city. Prevention was the only weapon health officials had for combatting the modern "plague." Citizens were advised to avoid crowds, cover their mouths when they coughed, and wash their hands, but the death rate grew.

In October 1918 Denver's health manager ordered churches and theaters closed and even "forbade" outdoor gatherings. Suddenly in early November fatalities decreased. On November 11, 1918, World War I ended and the health department retracted the restrictions. Thousands poured into the streets to celebrate the armistice, as the pall of violent death and destruction lifted. Then a second wave of illness struck. Deaths rose abruptly in late November, and bans were again imposed. But the public rebelled, refusing to eschew customary social events, and health officials withdrew orders to wear masks and close theaters and churches. The flu peaked the week of December 7, when 201 persons died, then it declined just as quickly.[71] Two isolation wards had been built in 1917, and Children's Hospital lifted its ban on contagious cases to admit flu patients. The annual report for 1919 cited a 4 percent death rate for flu patients, less than half the citywide rate.[72]

World War I and the flu pandemic opened the field of "infective diseases" within the hospital walls. In 1922 a smallpox epidemic brought a death toll in Denver of 270. The years immediately following the Great War also expanded orthopaedic surgery. The 1920s brought a new wave of children with bone tuberculosis, because some young soldiers sent to Fitzsimons Army Hospital with tuberculosis remained in the area and fathered children who in turn developed tuberculosis of the bone. Many of these patients ended up at Children's Hospital as charity cases. The disease involved the spinal column, hip, knee, ankle, and shoulder, in that order. Spinal and hip cases had lengthy hospitalizations. Dr. Robert Packard was first to perform spinal surgery, after which the child was fitted with a steel brace.[73]

In an era when the doctor-patient relationship was intensely personal, Dr. George Packard, Sr., made vivid impressions on many polio victims.

Four-year-old Anne Milavec was stricken with polio in 1920. Years later she fondly recalled the ministrations of Dr. Packard and the entire staff. She spent only a few weeks at Children's Hospital, where she was partially cured and fitted for a brace. The total cost of all treatment was $148.70.[74] Dr. Packard's sons also earned the patients' admiration. Clarinda Sewell contracted infantile paralysis at age seven. When Clarinda was not on her crutches, her back fell into an S curve. She spent two summer vacations at Children's Hospital, first for hip and foot surgery in June 1923, and a full plaster-of-paris body cast to straighten her back. In 1924 she had pioneering back surgery by Drs. Robert Packard and Hamilton Barnard. By 1926 she was walking. Dr. Packard had exerted a powerful personal force in her recovery. She was determined to walk "to repay the efforts of that dear Dr. Packard who had given so much."[75]

At Children's Hospital many cases were labeled simply as "infant feeding" problems, which comprised a large percentage of patient deaths. In 1920, 123 patients were diagnosed as such, with twelve deaths; in 1921 there were 125 cases with seventeen deaths. Some were likely premature births; others may have had surgical conditions not yet precisely identified. Dr. David Akers, who limited his practice to pediatric surgery, reported some "strange" diagnoses, including "autointoxication," "intestinal fermentation," "intestinal indigestion," and "intestinal intoxication." In 1926 out of forty-two cases of "intestinal intoxication," seventeen deaths occurred. Soon thereafter the diagnosis disappeared.[76] Other diseases also carried high fatality rates. In 1925 eighty-nine cases of influenza were treated, with thirteen deaths. Six of six meningitis patients died, as did thirty-four of ninety-one bronchopneumonia and fifteen of forty-three lobar pneumonias. Under the new category of "New Born," seven of ten infants brought in for "prematurity" died. Thus were introduced new definitions for problems of the newborn other than "infant feeding."[77] Handling premature infants would become an important hospital specialty long before neonatology evolved.

Young Seymour Wheelock's experience in 1923 at age five was more typical of Denver Children's Hospital patients. A reluctant candidate for T&A surgery, along with more than 1,300 other fellow patients operated on that year, he recalled repeated house calls to the family home by his pediatrician, Dr. Roy P. Forbes, followed by a humiliating, painful visit to Children's Hospital. Wheelock vividly portrayed the operation; he felt as if someone had "driven an enraged wildcat down his throat."[78] Given his early experience, it is perhaps remarkable that Wheelock would want to become a doctor. He recently completed a distinguished career of nearly forty years, first as a practicing pediatrician and later as director of Ambulatory Pediatric Medicine at Children's Hospital.

Just as the physician's world became more professionalized, so did that of nurses. By 1919 pediatric training was rapidly evolving at the Children's Hospital School of Nursing. Attrition remained a serious problem. Although only three of twenty-seven admitted were dismissed, sixteen pupils "severed connection with the Training School for various reasons." Fortunately the supply of nurses increased through hiring women trained elsewhere. In 1919 eighteen pupil nurses took training from St. Joseph's Hospital, twelve at Mercy Hospital, and two from Glockner Sanitarium in Colorado Springs.[79]

At Children's in the 1920s, professionalism was stressed. The superintendent of nurses emphasized technical and educational aspects of training above tight restrictions on social behavior and living circumstances. She noted that "many new features could be added to our course which would make it more attractive to young women who wish to take up nursing as a profession."[80]

The Class of 1921 was the first to serve all three years in the new facilities. Undoubtedly it was a challenging time for the nursing students. They experienced the war and the influenza epidemic together, as the latter claimed one of their number, Ellen Johnson. After graduation several continued their professional training elsewhere. Many enjoyed fascinating lives; Charlotte Crooks Leadmon was typical. Early in her marriage her husband died of pneumonia. She received additional training at Cook County Hospital in Chicago and worked at Letterman Hospital in San Francisco, joining the army in 1943. During the war she set up a hospital "from scratch" in England, where she was in charge of 2,500 sick and wounded German prisoners of war. Following D-day Leadmon was sent to Paris for more hospital work. After the war she became a free-lance artist.[81]

By 1920 many aspects of hospital management exceeded the abilities of amateur volunteers. Prewar and wartime inflation effectively doubled the cost of living between 1914 and 1920, and many Victorian-era board members had difficulty facing new economic realities. Professional accountants told the board that 8 percent of the workload for charity was all the association could handle, but it was running more than 10 percent, with

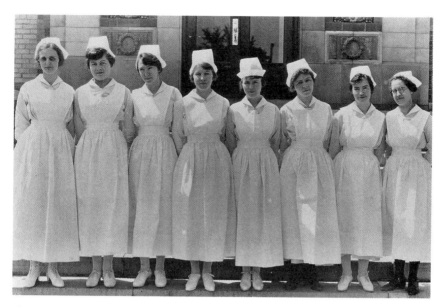

The Class of 1921, first to serve all three years in the new facilities. Pictured (left to right): Laura Freedinger, Pearl Strelow, Minna Kline, Catherine Ford, Lois Brandon, Winnie Argall, Hannah Richards, and Margaret Clark.

demand increasing relentlessly. By March 31, 1920, total assets reached $338,209.23. Children's Hospital Association members gradually realized the need to become more businesslike. While the board still welcomed gifts-in-kind such as food and blankets, they saw the necessity of concentrating on raising hard cash and endowments. Junior League gifts represented a transition from traditional to modern forms of female philanthropy. The league undertook the creation and support of a four-bed ward and aimed toward a fund of over $53,000 to maintain it.[82]

Fortunately, new philanthropists appeared at the threshold of the hospital's second decade. Harry H. Tammen, the publisher of the *Denver Post*, was romantically inclined; otherwise, one great source of future funding might not have evolved. Instead of presenting his wife a personalized gift, he handed her a check for $100,000 "for your string of pearls" a few days before Christmas. Children's Hospital was engaged in a fundraising drive of $50,000 for a new wing, and Mrs. Tammen had been asked

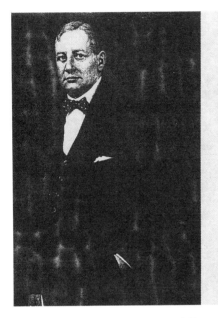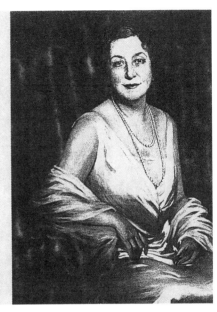

Harry H. Tammen and Agnes Reid Tammen, major benefactors whose Tammen Trust continues to provide for today's patients.

to donate $1,000. According to one source, she told her husband that it would be sinful to spend twice as much for personal pleasure than the entire wing would cost and asked if she could donate $50,000 for the proposed facility. Harry gazed fondly at his wife and replied: "You never cease to amaze me. We will give the entire $100,000."[83] Tammen soon doubled his contribution, and ground breaking for the Agnes Reid Tammen Wing was June 6, 1921.

The year 1924 marked a large transformation in scale and complexity at all organizational levels. A separate isolation ward was created in one of the four Ogden Street houses purchased by the association for about $27,000. A second house was used by the Junior League for a preventorium, another for a nurses' home (one of five in which the nurses were scattered). The last was rented to employees, yielding annual income of about $2,600.[84] Also that year Tammen placed $103,550.49 in the First National Bank in the name of "The Agnes and Harry H. Tammen Children's Hospital Fund," and for the first time Agnes Tammen's name appeared on the board of directors.

The Tammen Wing, costing about $200,000 with equipment and furnishings, opened on February 16, 1924, five months before the benefactor's death. At the opening ceremony Harry Tammen dedicated the wing "for a child's sake," which became the hospital's motto. The donors designated space and facilities for treatment of contagious and orthopaedic diseases, as well as the traditional social mission of a "sheltering home for foundlings."[85]

An Outpatient Department opened May 10, 1924, and served 3,238 patients its first year. Its purpose was decidedly charitable. The *Fifteenth Annual Report* noted: "At the clinics held in this department children of the worthy poor receive treatment at a nominal cost or entirely free of charge when unable to pay." The Outpatient Department treated many more patients than inpatient services for a fraction of the cost. In 1925 expenses for outpatients were about $10,500 out of a total of $145,400.[86]

Ironically the association suffered temporarily from the big Tammen bequest, as other potential donors shied away. The frontispiece of the annual report for 1925 stated that there was "a mistaken impression . . . that our recent large bequest is sufficient to cover the needs of our hospital. . . . We receive no financial aid from the Community Chest, the State, or the City and County of Denver, while in our Out-Patient Department we give service to hundreds of Denver's children irrespective of nationality, color or creed."

Once Tammen's estate was settled, however, the hospital had a sizeable nest egg. Tammen died in July 1924. He willed his house on Humboldt Street and one-half of his estate to Mrs. Tammen, who devoted much of her life to philanthropy for the hospital. After other gifts were bestowed, the Tammen will left the remainder to Children's Hospital as a trust fund in perpetuity. It amounted to about $2 million, and the trust yielded $100,000 to $200,000 annually for years. By the early 1990s the Tammen Trust Fund had increased to almost $18 million and yielded roughly $1 million annually for the treatment of indigent patients.[87]

By the mid-1920s pediatrics had emerged as a specialty in Colorado, with Children's Hospital its regional focal point. World War I, the influenza and smallpox epidemics, and school health programs all stimulated continuing growth of the institution. Admissions jumped to 2,636 inpatients

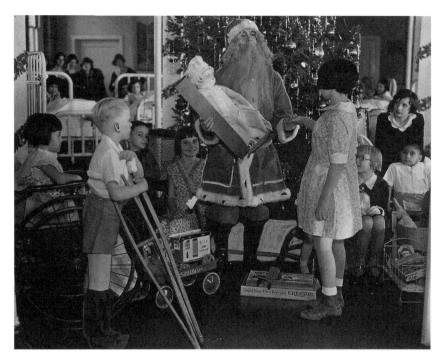

Santa Claus brought gifts to the hospitalized children.

and 3,238 outpatients in 1925. By then Dr. John Amesse was chief of staff
and Dr. George Packard, Jr., was secretary; thirteen pediatricians were
listed, including one woman, Dr. Elsie Pratt, who was the only woman on
the executive committee of the medical and surgical staff.[88]

The Tammen Trust expanded the traditional philanthropic and professional feminine spheres of endeavor in social services and the care of
indigent and low-income urban children. But the Tammen press lamented
that much more was needed. The trust fund opened a Pandora's box of
need. In 1924 the hospital had increased charity work fivefold from its first
year, but the need was never-ending. Only small reminders remained of
the highly personalized giving by the first women. Endowments of individual rooms still permitted donors to select the free occupants. Free beds
were contributed by benefactors, along with a record room and a fully

equipped laboratory. There were numerous additional individual gifts: a microscope, a microtome, a paraffin oven, and two baby scales. The Outpatient Department received gifts totaling $3,320 from several women, who also provided the salary of a social service worker. Mrs. Tammen apparently supported the female dental hygienist, and Mrs. Arnold Taussig and Mrs. Lawrence Phipps provided salaries for the hospital school instructor and set up the kindergarten.[89] The gifts of 1924 were a far cry from the domestic material goods provided to sick children by philanthropic women of the preceding decade.

In the "New Era" 1920s, women helped their professional sisters support social services and outpatient care that represented a greatly expanded community role for the hospital. By the middle of the decade Children's Hospital was unrecognizable when compared to the modest institution that had opened its doors fourteen years earlier.

Notes

1. "A Children's Hospital," *Denver Medical Times* 25 (1906): 27–28.

2. "Record of Proceedings," Preliminary Meetings of The Blanche Roosevelt Hospital for Children Association, April 5–July 5, 1906, CHD Collection; Robert W. Fenwick, "The 'Miracle' of Children's Hospital," in *Sunday Denver Post Empire Magazine,* September 12, 1965.

3. "Record of Proceedings," Preliminary Meetings, April 5–July 5, 1906.

4. Mrs. Alice Graham to Children's Hospital, October 2, 1912, CHD Collection.

5. "Record of Proceedings" Preliminary Meetings, April 5–July 5, 1906, 8.

6. Minutes of the Board of Directors, Children's Hospital, May 14, 1908; "Financial History of C. H.," 1906–1943, manuscript; both in CHD Collection.

7. Board Minutes, August 13, September 10, 1908; "Financial History of C. H."

8. *Rocky Mountain News*, June 19, 1908, reprinted in *Colorado Prospector* 5 (October 1974): 1; Board Minutes, November 3, 1908; "History of Organization," typescript from 1909 "Yearbook," CHD Collection; "Financial History of C.H."

9. Board Minutes, December 3, 1908, January 14, 1909.

10. Board Minutes, January 14, 1909.

11. "Embezzlement Charged to Society Woman," Denver *Times,* January 16, 1909, 1.

12. "Financial History of C. H."

13. Most financial information from "Financial History of C. H."; Board Minutes, August 11, 1909.

14. *Colorado Medical Journal* (May 1902): 226; "History of Organization," typescript, 1909 "Yearbook."

15. "Children's Hospital to Fight Attempt to Prevent Opening," Denver *News-Times*, November 28, 1909; "Fight on Children's Hospital Started by Residents," Denver *News-Times*, December 10, 1909.

16. Denver *News-Times*, November 28, 1909.

17. Stephen J. Leonard and Thomas J. Noel, *Denver: From Mining Camp to Metropolis* (Niwot: University Press of Colorado, 1990), 68; *Third Annual Report of the Children's Hospital and Training School for Nurses*, April 1911–April 1912, CHD Collection. The titles and form used for the hospital's annual reports have varied over the years. The time period of each report is from April 1 to either March 31 or April 1 of the next year. For consistency, annual reports are referred to here by the report number followed by the year it covers until the 1970s, thereafter by the year alone.

18. Denver *News-Times*, November 28, 1909.

19. *Second Annual Report*, April 1910–April 1911, 7.

20. Denver *News-Times*, November 28, 1909.

21. Unidentified clipping from Denver *News-Times*, ca. March 1910, CHD Collection.

22. Janet C. Cunningham, R.N., M.S., "Early Nursing, The Children's Hospital, Denver, Colorado; The First Decade, 1910–1920," n.d., typescript in possession of author.

23. Ibid.

24. *First Annual Report*, year ending April 1, 1910, 34–35.

25. *Second Annual Report*, 51.

26. *Third Annual Report*, 58–59.

27. *First Annual Report; Second Annual Report*, 8.

28. *Third Annual Report*, 15, 33.

29. Ibid.

30. Ibid., 19.

31. *First Annual Report*.

32. Quoted in Seymour Wheelock, M.D., "Starcraft, Leechlore and Wort Cunning," *The Children's Hospital, Medical Staff News* 1 (July 1990): 5, 7.

33. "The Children's Hospital," editorial in *Denver Medical Times* 29 (1910): 371.

34. *First Annual Report*.

35. Ibid.

36. *Second Annual Report*, 36.

37. Ibid.

38. *First Annual Report*.

39. *Second Annual Report*.

40. Herman I. Laff, M.D., "A Short History of Otolaryngology at Denver Children's Hospital," n.d. Laff's paper is part of a group of papers in the CHD Collection containing typescripts from former and present Children's Hospital physicians and medical department heads. Most typescripts were collected as part of an unfinished 1979 history project chaired by Edwin T. Williams, M.D., former president of the Children's Hospital medical and surgical staff. Some typescripts probably belonging to this group were not dated or identified. Other excerpts and segments of the hospital's medical history were parts of letters, reports, and speeches given by their authors. All of these are referred to hereafter as Physician Typescripts.

41. *Second Annual Report*; Charles Lockhart, M.D., "Anesthesia Department History," 1979, Physician Typescript.

42. *Second Annual Report*.

43. Ibid.

44. Wheelock, "Starcraft, Leechlore and Wort Cunning," 7.

45. *Second Annual Report*, Tables 1 and 2 on 22, 24.

46. *Third Annual Report*, 20–21; Clement A. Smith, *The Children's Hospital of Boston: "Built Better Than They Knew"* (Boston and Toronto: Littlo, Brown and Co., 1983), 64–69.

47. Laff, "A Short History of Otolaryngology."

48. *Second Annual Report*, 24.

49. *Third Annual Report*, 21; Richard A. Meckel, *Save the Babies: American Public Health Reform and the Prevention of Infant Mortality, 1850–1929* (Baltimore: The Johns Hopkins University Press, 1990).

50. *Second Annual Report*, 8–9.

51. Mrs. George Packard, Sr., *A Little Story of The Children's Hospital of Denver*, 7–8.

52. Ralph H. Verploeg, M.D., "Doctor of the Year," 1978, Physician Profiles, CHD Collection.

53. Hamilton I. Barnard, M.D., "Orthopedic Services at Children's Hospital, 1920 to 1940" and "Addenda to the history of orthopedics at Children's Hospital," probably 1979, Physician Typescripts.

54. Verploeg, "Doctor of the Year"; David Akers, M.D., "Preface" (to a surgical history), typescript probably written for the 1979 history, 5–6.

55. Verploeg, "Doctor of the Year."

56. Webb quoted in Leonard and Noel, *From Mining Camp to Metropolis,* 76, 79–80.

57. Barnard, "Orthopedic Service at Children's Hospital."

58. Ibid.

59. *Second Annual Report*, 17–18.

60. "Hospital Now Crowded," *Rocky Mountain News*, July 16, 1911.

61. Board Minutes, April 3, 1914.

62. Packard, *A Little Story*, 15–16; "Financial History of C. H."

63. "Ground Broken at Nineteenth and Humboldt," Denver *Times*, February 24, 1916.

64. "Tots Move to New Hospital," *Denver Post*, February 12, 1917.

65. Cunningham, "Early Nursing." Cunningham drew from the 1916 annual report for this.

66. *Seventh Annual Report* (1915–1916), 13–14; *Ninth Annual Report* (1919), 11–12; *Tenth Annual Report* (1920), 16–17.

67. *Eleventh Annual Report* (1921), 24; *Thirteenth Annual Report* (1923), 7, 21–22.

68. *Seventh Annual Report*, 13–14; *Ninth Annual Report*, 11–12.

69. Mabel G. Hodges to Board of Directors, in Board Minutes, April 7, 1920.

70. J. W. Amesse, M.D., *History of the Children's Hospital of Denver 1910–1947* (Denver, 1947), 53.

71. Katherine Anne Porter, *Pale Horse, Pale Rider: Three Short Novels* (New York, 1965), 232, quoted in Leonard and Noel, *Mining Camp to Metropolis*, 168.

72. James K. Todd, M.D., "History of the Division of Infectious Diseases at the Children's Hospital of Denver," n.d., Physician Typescript; Barnard, "Orthopedic Services at Children's"; *Ninth Annual Report*, 11.

73. Barnard, "Orthopedic Services at Children's."

74. Anne M. [Milavec] Slobko to Children's Hospital, ca. early 1980s, with bills attached, CHD Collection.

75. Clarinda K. Sewell to The Children's Hospital Foundation, January 9, 1986, CHD Collection.

76. Akers, "Preface," 4–5.

77. *Tenth Annual Report*, 32–33.

78. Seymour Wheelock, M.D., "Reflections on the 75th Anniversary of the Opening of the Children's Hospital," *Impact* (Summer 1985): 14–15.

79. *Ninth Annual Report*, 21.

80. Ibid.

81. Children's Hospital Association Alumnae Newsletter 16 (May 1968), CHD Collection.

82. *Tenth Annual Report*, 10, 12, 23.

83. Bill Hosokawa, *Thunder in the Rockies: The Incredible Denver Post* (New York: William Morrow and Co., 1976), 39–40.

84. "Financial History of C. H."; *Thirteenth Annual Report*, 4–9, 28, 29; Memorandum to Dr. Ed Williams from George L. Beedle, D.D.S., "The History of Children's Hospital Dental Service," 1979, Physician Typescript.

85. "Building of Tammen Wing of Children's Hospital to Be Started in Near Future; Site Is Purchased for $100,000 Addition Which Will Provide Facilities for Treating Contagious and Orthopedic Diseases and Care of Foundlings," clipping ca. 1921, probably from *Denver Post*, CHD Collection.

86. *Fifteenth Annual Report* (1925), 12.

87. "Financial History of C. H."; Mr. Len Dreyer, taped interview by Mark S. Foster, June 30, 1993.

88. *Fifteenth Annual Report*, 10.

89. "Children's Hospital Unable to Care for All Needing Help," clipping ca. December 1924, CHD Collection.

Chapter 3

The Hospital Takes Wings, 1925–1940

A local newspaper clipping on November 2, 1924, describing The Children's Hospital school for patients echoed the idyllic theme of almost three decades before at Dr. Love's outdoor hospital. "Quaint miniature furniture, enameled in flower hues," characterized Denver's "most unusual schoolroom," where sick children could "keep up" with their little peers in public school and "make their grade," even though hospitalized. "A low work table and tiny chairs give the youngsters a place to cut and paste and draw and paint to their heart's content." They make "baskets and mats and paper chains and posters and birdhouses and dolls." "A roof garden equipped with flower boxes, a gigantic dolls' house and a sand table also is very popular with the children."[1]

Mike Soltes, of Hungarian descent, was a special beneficiary of the hospital school. He was seven when his parents brought him to Children's Hospital in 1919 with a tubercular hip. His health was much improved a year later, and his parents took him to West Virginia where his father worked as a coal miner. Suffering a relapse, Mike was sent back to Children's and remained there more than two years. Over an eight-year period Mike returned to the hospital many times for care and treatment. His parents wanted him to return to West Virginia, but the board of directors feared he would suffer a relapse and lose all that he had gained. In a philanthropic tradition of noblesse oblige, they believed that because the parents had contributed less than $100 for his care, the board had the moral right to intervene. They took the case to nationally renowned juvenile court judge Benjamin B. Lindsey, who decided Soltes could remain until he was fourteen, then decide his own future.

Board president Carrie A. Kistler wrote to Agnes Tammen on August 20, 1931, reviewing the case and seeking funding for Mike's education through college and law school at the University of Denver. She told Mrs. Tammen that several women already were committed to Mike's welfare, and she recounted his considerable scholastic and civic honors at East High School.[2]

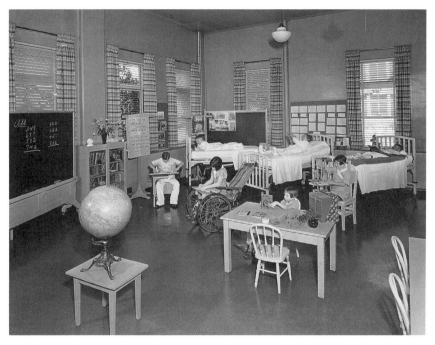

"School" came to the hospitalized children through the efforts of an educational committee assisted by Junior League members.

The school program at Children's Hospital symbolized the modern view held by its leaders of a hospital's very special role for children, because some of their young charges were likely to endure lengthy confinements. Growth and development — mental, emotional, educational, social, and physical — was a holistic concept. The school and other hospital departments sought to integrate the individual child into his peer group, family, and the larger community. The first members of the Hospital Association began planning a kindergarten in 1917; by 1921 organized lessons were taught.

From 1921 to 1931 most teaching was by Junior League volunteers. In 1925 there were fifty-nine pupils enrolled in classes, from age three to eighteen. In 1929 the Denver school board took over, and children received public school credit for completed work. Three years later public support was withdrawn because of the Depression, but the Tammen Trust supported private instruction. This arrangement continued until the Boettcher

School, connected to Children's Hospital by a tunnel under Downing Street, opened in 1940. Dr. Amesse reported proudly that, like Mike Soltes, many children subsequently went to colleges and universities. The educational program was a part of the hospital but not a detached one. According to Amesse, "It was rather a section of the whole plan for child care and guidance."[3] From 1932 to 1939 an average of eighty-six pupils enrolled every year, from kindergarten to twelfth grade.

The Boettcher School was largely a gift from Mr. and Mrs. Claude K. Boettcher, who donated $200,000 of a total cost of $388,000 toward its construction, in memory of his father, Charles Boettcher. The remaining funds came from a Public Works Administration (PWA) grant of $168,750, plus about $26,000 provided by the Denver Public Schools system.[4]

The 1920s marked a transition from the first-generation caretakers and trustees, as well as changes in the superintendent's role. At the turn of the century many hospital superintendents were women, with backgrounds in nursing administration or religious orders. They still were primarily caretakers, although they began to create national networks as did other groups of rising middle-class professionals in the Progressive era. The Association of Hospital Superintendents of the United States and Canada was founded in 1899 and renamed the American Hospital Association (AHA) in 1906. The AHA encouraged the scientific management of hospitals; by 1908 it had more than 450 members.[5] Mrs. Tammen and Oca Cushman toured leading facilities such as Massachusetts General and Johns Hopkins to study the managerial art.

In keeping with national trends modernization was a key issue addressed by new managers at Children's. The demands of scientific medicine made older converted domiciles and boarding homes inadequate. By the 1920s the Tammen Wing and other buildings made possible by the trust incorporated new technologies and more efficient operations. Superintendents had to balance the needs of the medical staff, patients, research, and teaching with rapidly escalating costs that philanthropy could not support alone. As the middle class occupied the majority of hospital beds, it also took on a larger share of hospital funding.

One historian notes that "the hospitalization of the middle classes changed the nature of the traditional institution as fundamentally as scientific medicine. . . . Doctors bore the primary responsibility for attracting these paying patients through referrals, but it was largely left to domestic

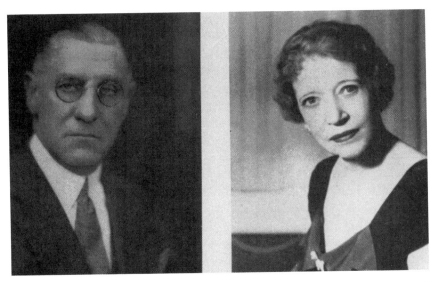

Mr. and Mrs. Claude K. Boettcher, who donated the funds for the Charles Boettcher School for Crippled Children. This was a Denver public school providing architecturally barrier-free facilities and an approved teaching program to children with physical handicaps, elementary through senior high school.

and nursing staffs under the superintendent's direction to adjust the day-to-day [operations] . . . to the care of middle-class patients."[6]

Oca Cushman personified the transition from the charitable and domestic values of the nineteenth-century superintendent to the modern, efficient nurse professional of the 1920s. She had attracted much of the early endowment, including the major share by the Tammens. She succeeded in this role until mid-century, through another generation of hospital managers and clinical practitioners. But many challenges in hospital organization and management and those of large-scale facilities expansion were taken over by Robert B. Witham of Rockford, Illinois. Like Dr. Amesse and many early physicians who brought health care west, Witham had a background in public health. He began as business administrator at Children's Hospital on October 1, 1927. On July 1, 1928, he was named director, and he served until November 30, 1937. He also prepared development plans for several buildings. Witham was succeeded by DeMoss Taliaferro, also from Illinois.[7]

Hospital records indicate that "divided authority" between Business Manager Witham and Superintendent Cushman dated from Witham's arrival in 1927. Evidence suggests that Mrs. Cushman yielded authority very reluctantly. For the next two years signs of conflict were noted among "Mr. W," "Mrs. C," the staff, and board. In 1929 there also was "great fuss among Mrs. Tammen, her lawyers and the board over what [is] charged to [the Tammen Trust] fund and how [the] hospital was managed."[8]

But Oca Cushman continued to monitor the minute details of patient nutrition and care. She carefully calculated "free, part-free, and full-pay" care by "patient days," as well as the diagnosis of each patient upon admission and the condition at discharge. Cushman's authority derived from the traditionally female-dominated spheres of nursing, domestic concerns, and social welfare services and was reinforced by the lay women board of directors. Witham assumed a traditional male role in business and management science, a role paralleling those of the fathers and husbands of many female trustees.[9]

Unbeknownst to its leaders Children's Hospital would face much greater challenges than the division of authority and accountability in the use of Agnes Tammen's generous gifts. Possible conflict over these issues was superseded by more general transformations in the larger socioeconomic environment of both the hospital and community. The bureaucratization signified by Witham's arrival challenged Oca Cushman's domestic management regime at the same time nursing was becoming more professional and complex. Witham in turn would be challenged by a new cadre of female professionals in nursing, social services, and physiotherapy.

The death of Harry H. Tammen in 1924 was a turning point in the hospital's history. The Tammen Trust, at the time valued at about $2 million, enabled the hospital not only to give free care to many needy children, but "to give to all the best care [and] to be able to contribute every facility for teaching and for research."[10] It also supported almost two decades of rapid expansion led by Agnes Tammen until her own death in 1942. Her activities symbolized the bountiful legacy of the hospital's first generation of philanthropists and physician founders.

By the 1920s most patients were from families able to afford their care. But the Tammen Trust enabled decision makers in the new Outpatient Department to continue admitting underprivileged children. The board instructed the staff that rates paid by families should ultimately be determined by the Social Service Department only after the patient was admitted and stabilized.[11] This policy relieved physicians of difficult decisions and removed the economic barrier in the doctor-patient relationship.

The Outpatient Department also initiated community outreach programs in the mid-1920s, beginning with a weekly nutrition class and "medical gymnastics" three mornings a week.[12] The department eventually conducted thousands of "home investigations." Dr. Amesse reported that it provided "encouragement, instruction and advice for the parents which might raise the standard of living in the family and in developing individualized post-hospitalization treatment plans."[13]

Children's Hospital remained a spiritual and spirited place, although religious imagery was more often replaced with the optimistic celebration of science, efficiency, and professional commitment. As its role in therapeutics and its commitment to care, education, and family support for the whole child evolved, professional social workers identified more with the medical staff than with the first-generation philanthropic women. As Dr. John Amesse noted, holistic health care for children was becoming more complex: "Medical social planning has included joint participation of the patient, family, doctor, nurse, often-times the occupational therapist, physiotherapist, dietician, administrative personnel and community agencies . . . whose services aided in physical restoration of the child."[14]

In 1930, because of Depression-era financial constraints, the Outpatient Department was closed. During its five years of existence, the department had examined 6,000 patients. While expressing hope that the department could be reopened in the near future, Director Witham noted that many patients would have to be referred to private physicians and community welfare institutions. He added that the department had experienced great difficulty in collecting fees, another reason for closure.[15]

Historians have argued that the hospital became a key middle-class institution nationwide in the 1920s. Hospitals emphasized the happy experiences of mothers and children inside their white, sanitary walls, where surgery became safe and acceptable. T&As, along with obstetrics, were the most popular fields for some physicians who depended upon paying patients. The "product" that hospitals offered to a new generation of "consumers" was the healthy newborn baby, a child cured of his or her diseased tonsils, a youngster avoiding the disaster threatened by a ruptured appendix, or a little patient scrambling around again after being felled by a broken bone.[16]

Increasing demand for preventive care for children meant that full-time careers could now be built on private practice. But it took time for pediatrics to be clearly differentiated from general practice. In 1920 more than three dozen medical schools in the United States and Canada offered training in child hygiene. Thirty-five leading pediatricians, including Drs. Gengenbach and Amesse, founded the American Academy of Pediatrics and established the American Board of Pediatrics as a national certifying body. The academy conducted its first national survey of pediatric practice in the late 1920s.[17]

When the University of Colorado Medical School established a Department of Pediatrics in 1930, school officials asked Dr. Gengenbach to serve as chair, a position he held until 1946. In the words of one anonymous historian, Gengenbach's commitment was "a harbinger of future relationships linking the community, the School, and Children's."[18]

The medical staff of 1926 had seventy-two doctors who rotated every three or four months to attend the "part-pay" and "gratis" patients in their sections. At that time physicians earned very modest fees, and some doctors attempted to bolster their incomes by other means. According to Dr. Gengenbach, many doctors engaged in the speculative mania of the late 1920s that preceded the stock market crash. He claimed that "all of the doctors were dabbling in the stock market," and were Republicans who believed in Herbert Hoover's promise of "a chicken in every pot." Brokers came to the hospital "peddling" stock. Gengenbach probably exaggerated the extent of speculation, but a surprising number of sophisticated medical specialists were quite innocent in dealing with financial matters. The following year the stock market crashed, and many fell upon hard times.[19]

At first the collapse affected only financiers; ordinary Denverites felt more gradual effects. From 1929 to 1932 the number of employed heads of households fell from 87 to 68 percent. In 1932 Denver mayor George Begole organized the city Emergency Relief Committee to coordinate Reconstruction Finance Corporation (RFC) loans and charity work, but the city would be bankrupt a year later. President Franklin Roosevelt's New Deal programs transformed public attitudes toward the widespread economic plight but provided only modest relief.[20]

The late 1920s saw a boom in hospital construction nationwide. Between 1925 and 1929 almost 80 percent more was spent on hospital building ($890 million) than in the previous four years. The real value of hospital construction in the late 1920s was not reached again until the 1950s.

Standardization and efficiency were predominant national values in the 1920s,[21] and Children's Hospital was no exception in its streamlining and specialization of the house and medical staff and building expansion.

Despite harrowing Depression-era economic and social conditions, Children's thrived. The material environment and optimistic spirit within Children's Hospital was a dramatic contrast to the plight faced by families outside. Thanks to the Tammen Trust and the dedication of hard-pressed community philanthropists, professionals, and staff, the 1930s was actually an expansive era for the hospital. Agnes Tammen supported an aggressive building program that acknowledged the professional status of nurses, social workers, and physiotherapists as well as the importance of treatment for paralysis and other crippling diseases of children.

The Agnes Reid Tammen Wing was built in 1931, providing additional orthopaedic beds; it also housed an auditorium, a patient library, and schoolroom. A new Department of Physiotherapy included hydrotherapy pools in the basement and a heliotherapy section on the roof. The 1936–1937 report recorded the opening of the hydrotherapy unit with two therapists and twenty-two patients on March 31, 1936; a year later there were eight technicians and from seventy to ninety patients daily. During the first year the department gave over 15,000 treatments.[22]

Operating costs for the hospital increased 22 percent from 1935 to 1936, the new physiotherapy program adding almost $90,000. Fortunately the Tammen Trust provided $262,607.31 for charity care, of which more than $13,000 was used to equip the new building. Mrs. Tammen also donated important gifts-in-kind: a Maximar X-ray machine, an elevator car, Christmas presents, and other items. A recreational and occupational therapy unit began with Junior League volunteers.

In 1936 hospital admissions totaled 3,311 children, the largest in its history. Yet board president Clara M. Van Schaack unrelentingly pushed for additional improvements, citing the continuing lack of accommodation for contagious disease. She recommended that the board and staff combine efforts to secure an isolation building to remedy this shortcoming.[23]

This challenge remained controversial. In late September 1936 the Executive Committee of the medical staff unanimously recommended to the board that acute poliomyelitis cases be admitted under "proper isolation." Polio was considered less infectious "than a number of entities now being cared for in this institution." But the board rejected the plea from the medical staff. In addition, the problem remained, as it had since 1910, of dealing with patients who developed contagious disease following admission. As early as 1910 the staff had formally recommended that a "stable" be converted to an isolation ward. The request was shelved, however, while the board considered plans for a new hospital. A decade later Dr. Amesse sponsored a similar initiative, with the same result.[24]

In response to a severe polio epidemic in 1937, the hospital finally renovated a house on Ogden Street to accommodate patients. Mrs. Tammen took more dramatic action. In early September she learned that there was only one iron lung in Denver, although two patients needed it desperately to stay alive. She authorized arrangements for immediate delivery of an iron lung to Children's Hospital at her expense. The Drinker respirator helped save the lives of children with paralysis of the chest muscles. It made the new Tammen Physiotherapy Wing the most fully equipped institution in the region for treatment of polio patients in the convalescent stage. President Franklin D. Roosevelt, a polio victim himself, sent a congratulatory telegram at the dedication of the wing.[25]

For all the drama associated with the polio epidemic, most sick children experienced the more common diseases. Statewide, in 1930 measles led with 12,312 cases, followed by mumps, 3,550; whooping cough, 2,257; chickenpox, 2,566; tuberculosis, 1,379; scarlet fever, 1,119; and diphtheria, 470. Smallpox was practically wiped out in urban Colorado, with only fourteen cases in Denver of 578 cases in the state. There were 232 cases of pneumonia statewide, but no deaths in Denver. The polio virus was latent that year, with only seventy-six cases in Colorado and fourteen in Denver. The state epidemiologist lamented that smallpox and diphtheria still caused needless suffering because all children were not vaccinated, and typhoid still showed sporadic outbreaks.[26]

At the national level, leading pediatricians stressed the social and psychological importance of growth and development of the well child. Wellness became a framework for the body of knowledge pediatricians required to oversee the health of American children, which began with the earlier focus on infant mortality. Children's Hospital still admitted only a small number of newborns, whose vulnerability generated the highest mortality rate among admissions nationwide.

Another strategy of wellness advocates was emphasis on parent education and preventive health care among the middle class. They launched an education campaign for mothers in infant feeding and hygiene. Babies and children were measured by newly established norms of

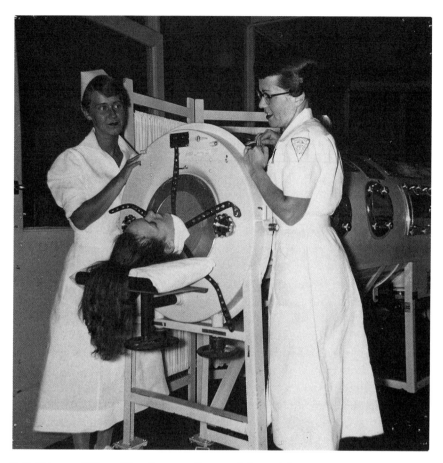

Polly Peterson, R.N., and Lou Shannon, director of physical therapy, visiting with patient in iron lung. Patients slept, ate, bathed, and exercised in the machines that did the breathing for their weakened chest muscles.

growth and development. Growth and development charts became the catechism of the new field of pediatrics. Through the decade, before the availability of effective sulfa drugs and biomedical technology developed during World War II, the formula laboratory remained as important as the pharmacy.[27]

The emergence of the specialty of pediatrics in the region was a great boon to the overall health of Denver families. Doctors reported that patients were often admitted in very serious condition. Dr. Max Ginsburg, the first resident at Children's Hospital, recalled that paying patients were admitted

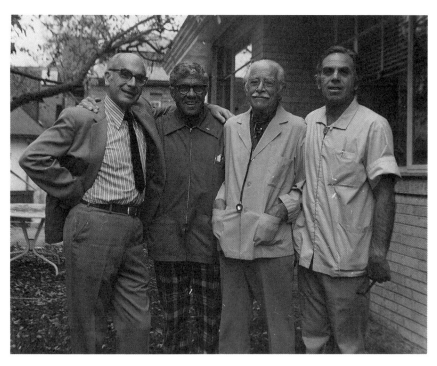

Dr. Max Ginsburg (third from left) was the first resident at Children's. He is shown here with Drs. Arthur Robinson, Leo Flax, and Jules Amer, associates in private practice in east Denver.

by private physicians not in family practice "who knew very little about treating children." Too frequently their charges had not even received preventive care until it was too late. The mortality rate for whooping cough was high, as it was in all hospitals. Tracheostomies were the "last resort," because there was no intensive care unit and patients could expel the tube if they were not under constant observation. The result could be fatal. Postoperative infections also were a complication. Doctors at Children's sometimes resorted to extreme measures. Dr. Ginsburg remembered a surgeon in a tuxedo doing a bedside emergency tracheostomy with his finger in the incision until a hemostat was found to keep it open. He then raced up the stairs, carrying the patient in his arms, in order to complete the procedure in the operating room. The patient recovered. Osteomyelitis was also common. A "new" treatment in 1928 was the application of maggots to untidy open wounds. This maneuver apparently had some positive effects, but the maggots sometimes escaped to unusual hiding spots, including other parts of the body. Many doctors at the time believed the treatment was a valid one, although Ginsburg called it "voo-doo medicine."[28]

In 1936 ninety deaths occurred out of 3,311 admissions at Children's Hospital, and in 1942 deaths numbered 107 of 4,444 patients. The largest number in both years was from pneumonia. New categories with high death rates appeared during these years, including congenital cardiac anomalies, carditis, and prematurity.[29]

Dr. Joseph Brenneman of the University of Chicago, who had trained several pediatricians at Denver's Children's Hospital, wryly warned that standardizing every aspect of the care and feeding of children and setting measurable standards of growth and development for each age was opening a Pandora's box. In 1931 he claimed in an article that

> when the scale and measuring rod became the sole arbiters of nutrition, and the height and weight charts became as fixed guides as if they too had been handed down on tablets of stone from Mount Sinai, . . . the natural effect on the mother when confronted by a standard was to proceed to standardize her child. . . . When his mother tried to coax and finally to force him to eat in order to bring him up to standard, as is done in the majority of homes, he either refused to eat or else vomited or dawdled over his meals for hours.[30]

Nevertheless, between World War I and World War II, the measurement syndrome permeated scientific pediatrics. Deviation of only 10 percent below or 20 percent above the mean marked a child as "abnormal." Psychosocial norms were also devised by Arnold Gesell and other experts in child psychology. In 1925 Gesell set down the minimum standards of mental health expressed by behavior. A White House conference committee report in 1932 surveyed research in intelligence testing, personality formation, language and motor development, and social adjustment.[31]

The interwar years brought profound changes to levels of training, performance standards, and working and living conditions for nurses across the nation and at Children's. More scientific training was beginning to take hold, but many hospitals were dominated by women like Oca Cushman, who devoted their entire lives to their profession. Yet many younger nurses became more demanding and less tractable or willing to accept long-term lifestyles bordering on the monastic.[32] Nevertheless change came slowly. Until the 1950s almost all hospital nursing schools required residence for student nurses. This implied a strictly regimented lifestyle for young women, who were largely separated from their families and the outside community.

As nurses gradually gained more professional autonomy, new techniques of scientific management emerged in nursing as in hospital administration and social work. In 1927 freshmen at the Children's Hospital School of Nursing began the summer with an intensive eighty-three-hour course in nursing procedures: fifty-eight hours in elementary nursing; ten hours each in hospital housekeeping and bandaging; and five hours in drugs and solutions. Total summer classroom work for the department was 269 hours, followed by work on the floors.[33]

In 1926 the *American Journal of Nursing* pointed to "a brief burst of enthusiasm" for rigid "procedures" that national leaders sought to standardize in all institutions. The effort was short-lived because of the constantly changing nature of medical care and the hundreds of varying procedures involved, along with diverse, strongly held opinions among doctors, patients, administrators, and the nurses themselves.[34]

Children's Hospital participated fully in the standardization mania while it lasted. In September 1926 the first director of nursing procedure was hired, Miss Bertha E. Rich, who boasted very impressive credentials: she had done recent postgraduate work at the Chicago Lying-In Hospital and had served as head of the Pediatric Department and instructor of pediatrics at the University of Minnesota School of Nursing, and as an instructor and supervisor of pediatrics of the Infant's Hospital of Milwaukee.[35] After coming to Children's Hospital, she instituted very specific new procedures on the Baby Floor. Among the "additions affecting nursing care" were glass cubicles, effective incubators, and a heated table in the "premature room." Director Rich lauded "a new type of restraint jacket which is comfortable and satisfactory and a device for closing in the top of the crib when the child needs freedom of movement but is too active to be left unguarded."[36] Clearly the era of liberal infant care had not yet arrived!

By 1932 the new orderliness attending nurses' training seemed to give way under the sheer expansion of facilities and the wide net cast for willing students. The Class of 1932 entered in two groups, eighteen in February 1929, another twenty-nine in September. Twenty-four eventually participated in the hospital's first formal capping ceremony.

Despite long hours, the young women found time for pranks and fun in every period. Class reporter Mary Gregg Snowden described life outside the wards and classroom, including initiation ceremonies in the Tammen

Wing Auditorium. "We were dressed in diapers and gowns, given breast milk from baby bottles, had to swallow oysters on a string, eat wieners from a bed pan and warm tea from urinals! Really! And crawl up and down stairs."[37]

Nurses' accounts from the period observed that, unlike their more pliable predecessors, the young women of the 1930s were outgoing and apparently difficult to control, even by the autocratic Oca Cushman and methodical Bertha Rich. Mrs. Cushman would have cringed had she known all of the girls' frolics in their Ogden Street abodes. But even Oca Cushman could not be everywhere at once. Snowden recalled:

> It was hard to cut capers but we managed! . . . cooking fudge and tomato soup at 3 A.M. And getting caught by Dr. Robert Packard shampooing your hair while the patients slept. Was it the table in Central Supply or really some other reason for the black eye that Ethel Brooks showed up with? Marylee Stahl ran a daily double with Bertha in hot pursuit — Marylee had stepped on Bertha's freshly scrubbed utility room floor on 1st South and Bertha was waving her mop — she was six feet tall but Marylee escaped![38]

The young women also enjoyed adventuresome sojourns outside Children's Hospital walls during their affiliation at Colorado General Hospital. There they had duty in the Outpatient Clinic and the OB-GYN Clinic, where they sometimes had to assist in home deliveries. "These always happened at night," Snowden remarked, "and took us to way down under the viaduct. Needless to say, some of the homes we went into were rather eerie." Slight risks also attended their ward service at Children's. One novice got her finger caught in an eclamptic patient's teeth at 5:00 A.M. Another was almost "shown the door" by a supervisor "when she became hysterical over the maggots she found in a bed."[39]

In the early 1930s Robert Witham took charge of planning a new nurses' residence, an urgent priority. At that time most professionals valued modern facilities; anything "dated" usually created a negative impression. Witham proclaimed the dispersed houses "absolutely unfitted for housing student nurses, in a deplorable state," with some constructed forty years before. They were old-style residences with each room converted for sleeping five to six girls. Bath and lavatory facilities were "most inadequate." Old lead-pipe plumbing was beyond repair, as were the crumbling foundations; heating was almost impossible. He surmised that

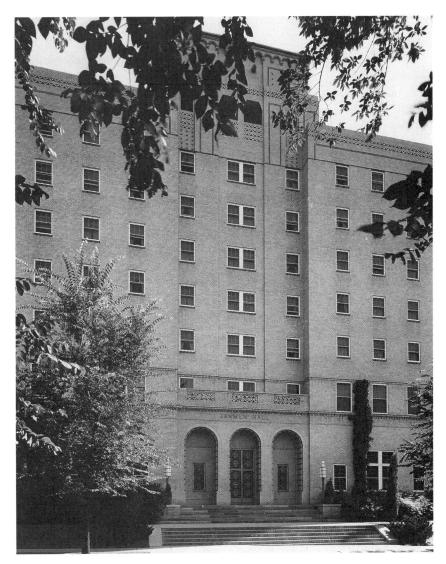

Tammen Hall, new nurses' residence completed in 1932; given by Harry Tammen to Children's Hospital in lieu of a set of pearls for his wife. Photo by Mile High Photo Co., Denver.

the city would have condemned them had Children's Hospital not occupied them.

Moreover, social opportunities for nurses were severely limited.
There were "no parlor facilities whatever in these buildings, and our
students are required to entertain their gentlemen friends on the street or
elsewhere," Witham lamented. He speculated that without the imminent
hope of a new home, not many would remain. Some students even donated
their monthly cash allowance of $8 toward the building.[40]

On December 11, 1930, Mrs. James C. Burger officiated at a dramatic
groundbreaking ceremony for Tammen Hall at East Nineteenth and Downing, a building costing approximately $300,000. Designed by architect
Merrill Hoyt, the building was light-colored brick like the main building.
Its eight stories contained 150 private rooms and baths for the nurses. The
main floor included a lounge, dining room, reception room, auditorium,
and offices. The basement held a well-equipped gymnasium with showers
and lockers. The second floor had classrooms, laboratories, a library, and
recreation rooms; the eighth floor, a roof garden and sunrooms.[41]

Tammen Hall, completed in 1932, was connected to the hospital
via a service tunnel. Its showcase was the first floor, symbolizing the
decorous social life of the young nursing students. Once inside the
vestibule, one entered a reception room. Across the hall was the large
auditorium. Off the main lobby was another reception room for men.
The west end of the corridor led to the main lounge — aesthetic and
modern in its appointments.

Sophisticated science was juxtaposed with the more traditional domestic luxuries now enjoyed by the student nurses. The second floor was
entirely given to education and contained a chemical and biological laboratory, fully equipped for teaching, and a dietetic laboratory. Oak tables
graced the labs and the library. Student rooms were uniform and modest,
each containing a paneled day bed, dresser, lounging chair, study table
with book-end compartment, an adjustable study lamp, and chenille material "harmonizing" with the color scheme.[42]

In 1932 the Nursing Service and School of Nursing were formally
separated through the appointment of Joy Erwin, B.A., M.A., R.N, as Dean
of Nursing. Erwin immediately tackled the vexing problem of the low
retention rate for Children's nurses. She explained why only twelve of
twenty-five recruits remained in the program nine months later. Five had
left from "lack of adjustment"; four "felt unsuited for the nursing profes-

sion, although they were good students"; two were "poor" in scholarship; one was getting married; and another was "needed at home." By 1939 turnover among nurse trainees had been reduced; nevertheless, less than 20 percent stayed more than two years. Because of the off-and-on status of the affiliation with the Colorado University's School of Nursing, many juniors went as far as the University of Minnesota. This may have influenced some nurses to pursue careers elsewhere. Others abandoned their careers when they married.

Dean Erwin took other reorganization measures. In the spring of 1939 an assistant dean for nurses was appointed. Other new personnel included clinical instructors for medical and surgical procedures, infant nursing, and orthopaedic nursing. These women supervised collegiate affiliation with the University of Denver.[43] Relatively few women became doctors, a condition that still characterizes the medical profession. Over a half-century later, when only 17 percent of all practicing physicians are women, an analyst at the National Institutes of Health (NIH) claimed that 90 percent of nurses in 1992 originally wanted to be doctors. She described nursing as "a distaff career track" for women interested in medicine.[44]

In 1940 every resident physician at Children's was male. Women had lost considerable ground on the medical staff. But nursing held strong as the most outstanding of the female professions at Children's, and the School of Nursing was accredited by the National League of Nursing Education. The dean announced completion of reorganization and the implementation of a five-year plan with Denver University for combined B.A. and R.N. degrees.[45]

Yet all was not well among the rapidly growing, diverse staff of health professionals, male and female. In 1937 an alleged sexual harassment and employment conflict developed between Mr. Witham and female physiotherapists. In a headline in early April, which sounds oddly contemporary, the *Denver Post* declared: "Denver Nurses Walk Out When Chief Is Fired; Six Also Protest Working Conditions at Children's Hospital; Afraid of Jobs." The next day another headline proclaimed the multiple internal tensions among female and male personnel at Children's.[46] Board president Clara Van Schaack was unsympathetic: "I think the girls acted hastily and will regret what they have done. There is not a chance of their being employed again at Children's Hospital."[47] The women who walked out were not nurses but members of the newer profession of physiotherapy, which perhaps had not yet gained complete acceptance as a suitable occupation for young women.

The young professional women reported scandalous, intolerable conditions of employment and claimed sexual harassment by Robert Witham. The board of directors, dominated by prominent women with Victorian moral standards, was clearly reluctant to address the charges directly. The board's Physiotherapy Committee acted decisively, however, to protect the hospital's reputation against both scandal and negativity among staff.

The committee stood even more firmly behind Director Witham — at least for the record. "It was brought to our attention," the committee wrote, "that Mr. Witham had been unduly familiar with the girls in the Department. The particular instance cited was not especially shocking, nor the evidence overwhelming. . . . we feel that if it were not for the feeling of antagonism against Mr. Witham, which had been spread by careful planning though the Department, that the matter would never have been reported, or seriously discussed."[48]

Significantly, the female professionals were disunited. The graduate nurses condemned the walkout as "disloyal and unethical." Superintendent Morrison emphasized that those who resigned "are not nurses. They have had specialized training in physical education and . . . hold college degrees, but they have not had nurses' training." She claimed: "No nurse would have done such a thing. All of our nurses are loyal to the hospital and they don't approve of walkouts." However, no hospital leader responded directly to the harassment charges. Fortunately for the physiotherapists involved, they were in demand elsewhere; apparently none experienced difficulty locating other positions. After the furor, a handwritten financial "history" of Children's Hospital noted, under the year 1937, that in June there was "Fuss over Physiotherapy dept. Mr. Witham left and Mr. T[aliafero] came."[49]

Just as professional training, work, and social conditions improved slowly for nurses during the 1920s and 1930s, so did they evolve for young resident doctors. Much of the training was informal, when they retained sufficient energy to catch the staff men on their rounds. The pay was not attractive. In 1928 Oca Cushman offered Dr. Max Ginsburg a residency at $100 per month. He bargained for $125 only because he had already completed a year's general training. Thus Dr. Ginsburg began a fifty-year career as a prominent Denver pediatrician. Significant staff additions dur-

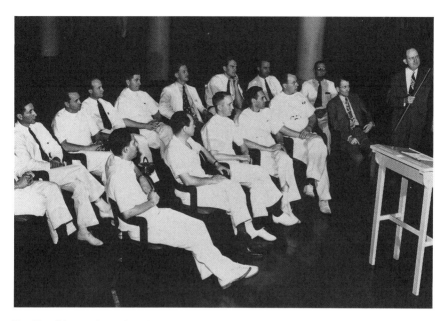

Dr. Harold D. Palmer, first full-time pathologist and medical director, teaching pediatric residents. Wayne Danielson, Ph.D., clinical chemist, is seated at the far left of the first row (ca. 1946).

ing the 1930s included Drs. Joseph H. Lyday and Ralph H. Verploeg. The latter was one of the first to have training in T&A surgery.

Children's Hospital was accredited for pediatric residency training in 1931 through — according to Lyday — Dr. Gengenbach's influence. In 1936 a two-year orthopaedic residency was approved, but surgical residency was not established until 1946. Until Dr. Harold D. Palmer arrived in 1942 as pathologist and medical director, young doctors had a "very informal" training program, and they endured night duty every third night.

Dr. Ginsburg had negotiated a comparatively munificent salary, but residents and interns worked long hours. Interns had one-half day off a week, and some received a monthly salary of $50 or less. Lyday recalled that "we were very busy but not very well satisfied. We were allowed to bring our wives for Sunday dinner without charge, courtesy of Mrs. Cushman. Yet, in those days an internship was an opportunity to apply one's medical school knowledge and to learn what one could from the attending staff physicians. The Chief Resident would attempt to set up programs for group teaching by staff doctors."[50] Still, instruction was catch-as-catch-can.

Living quarters for most house staff were in "Cannery Row," a six-unit row of small houses across from the present location of Tammen Hall. The staff had to pay for the coal for their furnaces. They ate family style at the hospital; one doctor recalled that fried rabbit was often the main course on Friday night. One advantage of residency was recreational. After the therapy pool was built, and if Oca did not catch them, the residents went swimming. An area behind the hospital facing Eighteenth Avenue contained a garden, weeping willows, and tennis courts. It eventually became a parking lot.[51]

Before 1934, when an "Accredited Staff" first was listed in the annual reports, only two men were assigned "on service" for specific parts of the year, with consultants on call at any time. Dr. David Akers noted that "the burden was not very onerous" because of the small number of surgical cases. By 1934, 191 physicians were listed on the accredited staff, including at least forty-four surgeons.[52] These seemingly impressive numbers probably demonstrated the extreme glut on the professional market during hard times. Being listed on The Children's Hospital staff unquestionably brought ego satisfaction to many physicians with a dearth of paying patients. Very few women physicians served.

Nevertheless women dominated nonmedical hospital departments, including some important positions on the house staff. A registered nurse managed the Formula Laboratory, filling "milk prescriptions," and resident physicians occasionally tested new formulas there. These preparations augmented human milk. Women also handled a new medical records room established in 1936, although it was poorly staffed in the early years. In 1938 it had one secretary in charge who also took surgical dictation. Responsible physicians were requested to summarize each hospital chart in handwriting. Chart numbering and cross-indexing systems made it easier to review cases and conduct research.[53]

Dr. George S. Frauenberger was hired in 1938 to improve specialized physician training. Most patients admitted were curable and benefited from the latest advances in therapeutics and treatment, mostly in orthopaedics and improvements in the T&A procedure. Outpatient services existed for orthopaedics, physiotherapy, and occupational therapy. By then a dental clinic and an eye clinic also had been established. Residents rotated through the pediatric outpatient departments at Colorado General and attended well-baby clinics once a week. Dr. Frauenberger stayed at Children's Hospital only one year.

Unfortunately, during the 1920s and early 1930s rudimentary, even primitive therapeutics in vital specialties were still utilized by some staff physicians. Years later Dr. Lyday claimed that 90 percent of deaths in the hospital in the mid-1920s could have been prevented by today's standards. The majority of deaths through the mid-1930s were from gastrointestinal disorders and infectious diseases. The majority of admissions, however, were for T&A surgery, with small risk.[54]

Otolaryngologist Herman I. Laff reported that in Denver during the Depression, T&A surgery was prized by pediatricians and general practitioners. Some otolaryngologists charged $100 to do the procedure, a huge fee for the 1930s. Older pediatricians regularly encouraged younger physicians to undertake the operation, not the "fashion" in other large cities, according to Laff. This created "quite an undercurrent of displeasure" among the younger local specialists.

Laff claimed that Denver doctors often made a common medical error, causing complications by unrestricted use of nasal drops and sprays. Instrument size hampered progress in timely diagnosis of pulmonary tuberculosis. Pediatricians resisted examining small patients with full-sized instruments for fear of damaging their bronchial trees, thus missing the opportunity to diagnose some of the other diseases of the small bronchi of infants.[55]

Medical investigators clearly needed to develop smaller instruments and dosages more suitable for infants and small children. Administering intravenous fluids became a matter of life and death. In the mid-1920s techniques were usually crude. Doctors usually "pushed" these in all at once, according to one practitioner. Dr. Ralph Verploeg recalled modifications of scale in dosages and smaller instruments used for early training in Chicago for T&A surgery, subcutaneous infusions of premature infants, peritoneal injections, and "cut-down" I.V.s. But widespread change was gradual. Lyday remembers "run-away" fluids, overhydration, and the "problems of adult equipment for tiny people." When Dr. Wayne Danielson (Ph.D.) arrived at Children's Hospital, he initiated important research in the area of pediatric microbiochemistry.

In March 1933 Bertha Rich, director of nursing procedures, jubilantly noted in her report to the board:

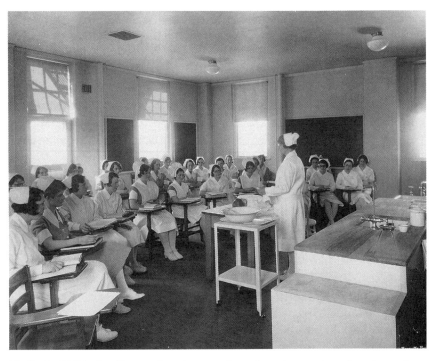

Ms. Bertha E. Rich, first director of nursing procedures, lecturing to a class of nursing students in Tammen Hall.

> Among life-saving treatments used here FOR THE FIRST TIME in the past year should be mentioned the continuous venoclysis. This is a method of supplying fluid and nourishment that cannot be tolerated by the usual route directly into the vein. New babies with summer diarrhea whose lives had been despaired of were restored by this treatment. In November and December, 76 patients were admitted with pneumonia; only thirteen died.[56]

Nationwide, medical research saw other key advances in the 1930s. The mysteries of the gastrointestinal tract gradually became sorted out with the recognition of deficiencies, chemical and protein imbalances, allergies, and the role of infection. By 1938 the death rate from gastrointestinal disease was greatly diminished, but reducing mortality rates in infectious diseases was only beginning.

In the mid-1930s, influenced in part by the fact that President Roosevelt was afflicted with the disease, public health policymakers promoted increased government support for polio management and research.

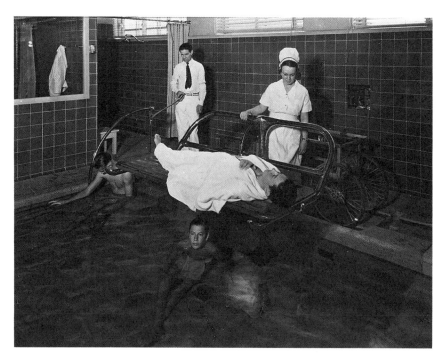

Hydrotherapy pool located in Agnes Reid Tammen building. Hydraulic lifts were the invention of Fred Hart, dairyman from Longmont, whose grandson was a patient in the hospital.

A 1934 study by two Colorado agencies found a thousand children needing treatment. The State Board of Health reported that faster identification of needy children and more facilities were required. Many youngsters suffering correctable disabilities of long standing were not rehabilitated because of lack of funds. The National Foundation for Infantile Paralysis provided some support. Special appropriations to the states also were designated by the Social Security Act of 1935. The State Board of Health used these funds to create the Division of Crippled Children, in time to oversee the polio epidemic of 1937. Two women with affiliations at Children's headed the division: Dr. Vera H. Jones as director and Marie Wickert, a social worker, as assistant director.

In early 1936 the hydrotherapy addition to the Agnes Reid Tammen Wing was completed. It contained a large treatment pool, primarily for patients with infantile paralysis; a "hot" pool kept at 100 degrees for polio cases emerging from the acute stages; and a chemical or "salt" pool for special infections such as tuberculosis of the bone, arthritis, and osteomyelitis. The upper floors had protected sun terraces at each level. Mrs. Tammen paid attention to detail down to the color scheme, with a view to the child's emotional response as well as physical therapy.[57]

Numerous recent inventions aided patients. Fred Hart of Denver designed a special hydraulic lift especially for Children's. The department also incorporated whirling arm and leg baths, hydrotherapy, shortwave therapy, infrared, ultraviolet rays, radio shortwave, muscle testing, and other corrective devices.[58] These pools are now storage areas.

Despite significant expansion hospital occupancy remained very high in the late 1930s. President Clara Van Schaack noted that "because of the continued unemployment causing disease and malnutrition among children, the demand for free and part-pay hospitalization is still extremely high." In 1935 over half of all children admitted received charitable support. The Tammen Trust contributed over $212,000, an increase of 59 percent over its support the previous year. In 1936 Tammen assistance increased another $50,000.[59]

The greatest epidemic of infantile paralysis in Colorado occurred in 1937. Immediate care was essential to limiting residual paralysis. The State Board of Health claimed that of 237 local cases reported, almost every child was treated rapidly and effectively, greatly reducing the extent of permanent crippling. Further treatment was given to sixty-four paralytic cases under age twenty-one. But the state also estimated 2,000 untreated crippled children in rural Colorado. Program demands would increase over the next several years, as parents and hospitals dealt with the residual effects for children with permanent disabilities.[60]

The transition from the hospital as a women's sphere, with most therapeutics based on traditional domestic care, to a more depersonalized scientific institution dominated by both male and female professionals, occurred within the first generation of hospital founders. This was accompanied by parallel expansion in professional roles dominated by women: nursing, social work, and certain therapeutics, notably physiotherapy and rehabilitation.

Leaders at Children's Hospital modernized both the equipment and the delivery of new medical procedures, but many of their functions were still of a traditional, nurturing character. Dietary and nursing care remained the largest patient care expenses, signifying continuity from the old to the new Children's mission, and its nurturing role in the community. In

1937 the Education Committee reported the largest pupil attendance in the history of the hospital school, with forty-two in junior and senior high and sixty in the elementary grades.[61] Attention to the whole child remained a consistent, unwavering vision as the first-generation supporters passed the torch to the second.

The growth of the house and medical staffs, plus statistics on admissions and deaths in the 1920s and 1930s, show the geometric expansion and growing complexity of the entire hospital organization. In 1926 doctors and surgeons were still almost entirely men, while women professionals were clustered on the house and nursing staff. In 1930, of three resident physicians one was female.[62] The hospital retained the mix of strong personalities and feeling of personal dedication conveyed by the directors, nurses, and physicians. A new cadre of business administrators, social workers, and physiotherapists greatly expanded the hospital bureaucracy. The late 1930s also brought an overturning of the traditional structure of hospital authority. The professions of pediatric nursing, social work, education, and occupational and physical therapy were newly emergent female spheres, which somewhat balanced the male-dominated medical and surgical staff.

The focus on development and health of the individual child, not just his or her physical problems, was consistently evident in the annual reports. Like their public health counterparts, pediatric nurses perceived their integral function as caring for the whole child. Prevention and holistic care were as important as curative medicine in Children's Hospital.

Historian Barbara Melosh notes that the mission of "positive health" linked visiting nurses associations, settlement houses, child welfare, and antivenereal disease associations in a common endeavor that extended well beyond hospital walls and the mostly male medical profession. The first female physicians at Children's demonstrated this orientation, as did its newly emerging departments in social services, education, and therapy. Beginning with the Sheppard-Towner Act in 1921, maternity and infant care programs became the "backbone of public health in the 1920s." By the end of the decade, nearly every state had prenatal and infant care programs. These programs dominated public health nursing through the 1930s.[63]

As nurses joined the ranks of new female health and welfare professions, they assumed the profile of "experts" rather than fitting into domestic traditions of "womanly service," with moral and religious connotations. Scientific method replaced intuitive skills, nurturing, and sympathy as the prerequisites for professional status. Leaders promoted separation of ward service from nursing education, seeking theoretical knowledge through colleges and universities rather than hospitals. Despite reformers' efforts, however, the "ideology and culture" of the hospital schools remained "at the center" of nurses' "distinctive craft culture," until the 1970s and beyond. As late as 1974 more than three-quarters of all active nurses obtained diplomas from the hospital schools.[64]

In 1936 nursing director Bertha Rich still conveyed familiar traditions of care in the Baby Department. Her report portrayed a peaceful, timeless scenario in the midst of the biotechnological flurry surrounding the new addition. The only equipment depicted as sophisticated were the electric humidifiers. Her 1936 report also belied the perception of her original role as procedural efficiency expert. Miss Rich's phraseology was emotional, attributing health to traditional domestic nurturing and affection rather than science. She described the "serene, happy environment" vital to the welfare of the "very sensitive" babies, "unable to tell by the usual language when something is wrong." The smaller infants required "more than usual vigilance" to prevent even slight infections such as the common cold, which could become critical. Each baby was thus "kept from direct contact with every other person. He has his own individual equipment, including a sterilized bath tub. The nurse's hands are always freshly washed before she comes to him, and he is picked up with his own quilted pad to protect him from contact with her uniform." She emphasized importance of the feeding procedure, natural air, and light to infant survival and vitality.

> At feeding time, each baby is gently awakened and held comfortably in the nurse's arms. This "conditioning" the infant to his meal has been proved . . . to have an important bearing on the nutritional progress of babies. . . . He soon learns to feed himself, while the nurse is near at hand to help if he grows tired. . . . Daily weather permitting, all who are not acutely ill are taken into the outdoor sunshine. . . . When awake, these babies hear low voices talking to them, much as they might at home. Long before a baby understands words, he is responsive to the tone of voice and is sensitive to the behavior of adults.[65]

But there also were many "desperately ill babies to be cared for." Miss Rich stressed the critical importance of efficient and safe procedures in infant care. Then as now, the work was very labor-intensive. Nursing care of a single convalescent baby demanded almost eight hours a day, under the "sole attention of one nurse."[66] Obviously, close attention had to be paid to recovering infants around the clock.

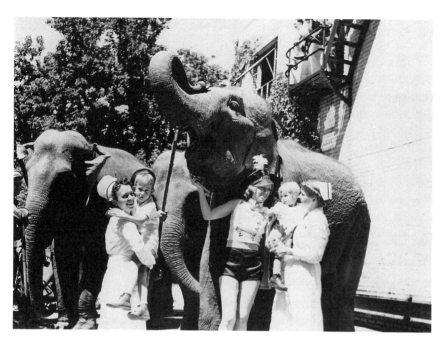

Entertainment came to the hospitalized patients in many forms, particularly when the "circus came to town."

In 1937 Miss Rich became nursing arts instructor, and scientific instruction overtly superseded "procedure" in the School of Nursing curriculum. There were 180 nurses at Children's Hospital: eighty-three graduate nurses, twenty-three affiliated, fifty-eight students, and twelve postgraduates for special courses. Tammen Hall was initially filled with first- and second-year students; many juniors left for affiliated work in adult nursing at the Colorado State University Hospital, or psychiatry in the Colorado University Psychopathic Hospital. The University Hospital School of Nursing reopened in the fall of 1936, when Children's reestablished affiliation.[67]

By the mid-1930s hospitalization was a common occurrence for children, with an estimated one out of every twenty-four children in larger cities becoming a hospital patient. Almost a third of pneumonia cases were hospitalized. Over half the children admitted were for surgery, with T&As the most common procedure. As the Depression subsided in the late 1930s, hospital use expanded, with occupancy rates for general hospitals rising from 64 percent in 1935 to 70 percent in 1940, considerably below Children's Hospital of Denver. Still, nursing and technology such as the orthopaedic facilities at Children's were the only treatments available for most infectious disease, paralysis, and congenital conditions. Scarlet fever required careful nursing to avoid its frightening complications. A ruptured appendix could result in peritonitis, which carried a high mortality rate. Pneumonia required carefully regulated body temperature, daily enemas, alcohol sponges, strapping the chest, sedatives, aggressive serum treatment after laboratory analysis and diagnosis, and oxygen therapy. These procedures saved many children from permanent disability.

Most infectious diseases had no effective cure before the advent of the drug sulfanilamide in 1937. Rather, the battery of labor-intensive procedures was all that might keep the patient alive through a crisis. One author has observed that a case of typhoid fever managed today by the best methods available in 1935 would require a hospital stay of perhaps fifty days, with minute attention to diet, daily laboratory monitoring, and possible abdominal surgery in a crisis.[68]

Within three years of the appearance of the sulfa drugs, however, intense nursing care was supplanted by medical specialization. By 1940 nearly a fourth of all practicing U.S. physicians were full-time specialists and many more were part-time. The hospital was a necessary "technological center" for diagnostic services in X ray and pathology, for surgery, anesthesia, as well as expert twenty-four-hour nursing care.[69] As World War II loomed, The Children's Hospital was poised to participate actively in the next generation of advances in medical care for young patients.

Notes

1. "Children in Hospital Study to Maintain School Grades," November 2, 1924, unidentified clipping in CHD Collection.
2. Carrie A. Kistler to Agnes Tammen, August 20, 1931, CHD Collection.
3. John W. Amesse, M.D., *Children's Hospital; A History of Achievement and Progress From 1910 to 1947* (Denver, 1947), 83–88.
4. Ibid., 65.
5. Morris J. Vogel, "Managing Medicine: Creating a Profession of Hospital Administration in the United States, 1895–1915," in Lindsay Granshaw and Roy Porter, eds., *The Hospital in History* (London and New York: Routledge, 1989), 243–260.
6. Vogel, "Managing Medicine," 247.
7. Amesse, *Children's Hospital*, 31–32.
8. "Financial History of C. H.," 1906–1943, manuscript, CHD Collection.

9. The idea of parallel spheres of authority and the changing roles in hospital management is from Vogel, "Managing Medicine," 250–251. For a sketch of Cushman see Amesse, *Children's Hospital*, 31.

10. *Sixteenth Annual Report of The Children's Hospital Association* (1926), 12.

11. Board of Directors to the Staff, including "Rules for the Admission of Part-Pay and Charity Patients," June 27, 1925, CHD Collection.

12. *Sixteenth Annual Report*, 36.

13. Amesse, *Children's Hospital*, 81.

14. Ibid., 81–82.

15. *Twentieth Annual Report* (1930), 11, 17, 45.

16. Rosemary Stevens, *In Sickness and in Wealth: American Hospitals in the Twentieth Century* (New York: Basic Books, Inc., 1989), 106–108, 382, n.1. Statistics on hospital admissions from Selwyn D. Collins, "Frequency and Volume of Hospital Care for Special Diseases in Relation to All Illnesses Among 9,000 Families, Based on Nationwide Periodic Canvasses, 1928–1931," *Public Health Reports* 57 (September 25, 1942): 1447, table 8. Collins also reports that by 1930, 80 percent of all surgical cases were hospitalized, although over 90 percent of all nonsurgical conditions were still cared for in the home. See Stevens, 382, n.1, from Collins, "Sickness and Health: Their Measurement, Distribution and Changes," *Annals of the American Academy of Political and Social Science* 237 (January 1945): 153–163.

17. Sydney A. Halpern, *American Pediatrics: The Social Dynamics of Professionalism, 1880–1980* (Berkeley: University of California Press, 1988), 92–95; Al Miller, "The Sands of Time" (history of staff through the 1950s), n.d., Physician Typescript.

18. "A Brief History of the Department of Pediatrics, University of Colorado Medical School," ca. 1993, typescript, CHD Collection.

19. "Physician Memories," December 1984, Physician Typescript, CHD Collection, 1–2.

20. Stephen J. Leonard and Thomas J. Noel, *Denver: From Mining Camp to Metropolis* (Niwot: University Press of Colorado, 1990), 203–214.

21. Stevens, *In Sickness and in Wealth*, 148.

22. *Twenty-seventh Annual Report* (1937), 16.

23. *Twenty-seventh Annual Report*, 17.

24. "Re: Contagion," typescript of Board Minutes from November 28, 1910, through September 23, 1937, CHD Collection. Apparently these were checked and compiled for the board deliberations relating to the polio epidemic.

25. "Iron Lung Donated," *Denver Post*, September 28, 1937; "Denver's Children Share Top Medical Facility," *Rocky Mountain Herald*, May 4, 1974, 1.

26. *Annual Report of the Colorado State Board of Health* (Denver: State Office Building, 1930), 11–15.

27. Rickey L. Hendricks, "Feminism and Maternalism in Early Hospitals for Children: San Francisco and Denver, 1875–1915," *Journal of the West* 32 (July 1993): 61–69.

28. "Physician Memories," December 1984; Dr. Max Ginsburg to Mrs. Marion Fisher, March 14, 1991, CHD Collection.

29. Joseph H. Lyday, M.D., "Medical Progress at Children's Hospital, 1924–1942," Physician Typescript, 9–13.

30. Joseph Brenneman, M.D., "The Menace of Psychiatry," *American Journal of Diseases of Children* 42 (1931): 384–387, quoted in Halpern, *American Pediatrics*, 107.

31. Halpern, *American Pediatrics*, 88–89.

32. *Sixteenth Annual Report*, 29.

33. *Seventeenth Annual Report* (1927), 39–40.

34. Barbara Melosh, *The Physician's Hand: Work, Culture and Conflict in American Nursing* (Philadelphia: Temple University Press, 1982), 173–175.

35. *Seventeenth Annual Report*, 39–40.

36. *Eighteenth Annual Report* (1928), 41.

37. Children's Hospital Association Alumnae Newsletter 16 (May 1968), CHD Collection.

38. Ibid.

39. Ibid.

40. Robert B. Witham to President and Chairman of the Board of Directors, "Report of Investigation Covering Nurses Home," ca. early 1930, CHD Collection.

41. "Nurses' Home Started," *Denver Post*, December 11, 1930.

42. *Twenty-second Annual Report* (1932), 25–26.

43. *Twenty-eighth Annual Report* (1938), 27–29; *Twenty-ninth Annual Report* (1939), 28.

44. "A Cure for Sexism," *U.S. News and World Report* 112 (March 23, 1992): 86.

45. *Thirtieth Annual Report* (1940), Historical Number for Thirtieth Anniversary, 29–30.

46. Ben M. Blumberg, "Denver Nurses Walk Out When Chief Is Fired," April 4, 1937, *Denver Post;* "Nurses Assail Walkout Here," April 5, 1937, *Denver Post.*

47. "Denver Nurses Walk Out."

48. "The Physiotherapy Committee present the following report," April 8, 1937, typescript, CHD Collection.

49. "Nurses Assail Walkout Here"; "Financial History of C. H."

50. Lyday, "Medical Progress."

51. "Physician Memories," December 1984, 2, 4.

52. David Akers, M.D., "Preface" to a surgical history, typescript probably written for the 1979 CHD history, 6.

53. Miller, "The Sands of Time," 10a.

54. Lyday, "Medical Progress," 10.

55. Herman I. Laff, M.D., "A Short History of Otolaryngology at Denver Children's Hospital," typescript in 1979 CHD history, 4–5.

56. *Twenty-third Annual Report* (1933), 27.

57. Untitled typescript history, ca. 1935, CHD Collection; *Twenty-fourth Annual Report* (1934), 14; *Twenty-sixth Annual Report* (1936), 14–15, 26, 32; Amesse, *Children's Hospital,* 73; Report and drawings, "Master Facilities Project," Haller & Larson Ltd. Architects, 1917–1982, CHD Collection.

58. *Twenty-sixth Annual Report*, 14–15, 26, 32.

59. Ibid.

60. *Annual Report of the Colorado State Board of Health* (Denver: State Office Building, 1937), 14–19; Table, 42.

61. *Twenty-seventh Annual Report*, 16–17, 37, 39, 42.

62. *Twentieth Annual Report*, 11–12.

63. Melosh, *The Physician's Hand*, 113–120. Melosh states that public health professions moved Progressive reform from "moralism to pragmatic environmentalism. . . . As epidemics swept through one city after another, concerned citizens worked to identify and control the sources of infection. Before the elaboration of the germ theory, many observers concluded that disease was spread by miasma, the insalubrious airs exuded by garbage,

open sewers, and overcrowded districts." Associations that became involved in this movement included the antituberculosis associations that funded educational efforts. A national association began in 1904 with chapters in Baltimore, Cleveland, and Chicago. Public health reformers also focused on the home and family, marked by the 1909 White House conference on infant and maternal health.

64. Ibid., 119–120.

65. *Twenty-sixth Annual Report*, 47–48.

66. Ibid.

67. Ibid, 35–37.

68. Dr. Seymour Wheelock, telephone interview by Mark S. Foster, June 24, 1993. Treatment with chloramphenical, an effective antibiotic, has reduced the mortality rate for typhoid fever from about 20 percent to 1 percent and the length of a hospital stay to as little as a week.

69. Stevens, *In Sickness and in Wealth*, 172–173.

Chapter 4

World War II and Peacetime Growth, 1940–1958

The upheaval in physiotherapy in 1937 and the sudden departure of Witham were symptomatic of the major social, professional, and medical changes that took place inside hospital walls through World War II and the succeeding decade. The mid-century years brought immense challenges to the hospital and all personnel. Not only did physicians and other high-profile individuals associated with Children's reap greater publicity for their contributions to health care and the advancement of scientific knowledge, but all hospital workers enjoyed a greater sense of professional identity by the end of this period.

After years of only moderately successful economic experimentation by the federal government, the Depression ended abruptly, largely because of wartime mobilization. In September 1939 Germany invaded and conquered Poland, beginning World War II. Through the Lend-Lease Act, which ultimately gave $51 billion in supplies and aid for the anti-Axis nations, the United States entered the conflict in all but military engagements. Hospitals faced a new challenge—severe shortages of supplies and personnel for the duration of the war. In 1940, a full year before the United States entered the conflict, Director Taliaferro concluded that Children's Hospital needed to cut drastically the admissions of charitable cases. He advised physicians, the general public, and "all referring agencies" that "this hospital does not accept the ordinary indigent case." State and municipal facilities would have to care for medically indigent children, with Children's accepting them only in emergencies.[1]

World War II saw dramatic advances in medical knowledge, particularly therapeutics, based on knowledge gained in the previous decade. In 1936 investigators from Johns Hopkins University had administered an experimental sulfa drug to President Roosevelt's son, who was suffering from a severe streptococcal infection. This medical success was in dramatic contrast to the death of President Coolidge's son twelve years earlier from blood poisoning resulting from a tennis blister on his heel. Before the introduction of sulfonamides, blood poisoning struck terror in parents' hearts. Suddenly drug companies could provide "magic in a bottle." Clinical reports in the U.S. medical literature regarding sulfanilamides, first published in 1937, heralded a dramatic new cure for pneumonia. Within a decade patients with pneumonia were elevated in medical texts from the most difficult cases to treat to "one of the simplest examples of therapy a hospital intern meets." Septicemia, meningitis, gonorrhea, dysentery, and chronic bladder infections were treated far more effectively with the new drugs.[2]

Penicillin was discovered in Britain in 1928, but its potential for curing diseases remained undeveloped until World War II. A critical reason was lack of knowledge on how to create a supply. In 1942 there was only enough penicillin worldwide to treat a single case! The Office of Scientific Research and Development (OSRD) sponsored a massive expansion effort, however, spurred largely by prospects of saving wounded soldiers' lives. Like so many other government-sponsored emergency efforts, this succeeded beyond expectations; by the end of World War II penicillin was available to the general population. The war greatly stimulated medical research in the United States and launched the great era of federal funding for biomedical research in the following decades. By 1947 half of all drugs in use had been developed within the previous decade.[3]

Health studies of the U.S. military pool indicated other areas for concern. The major health problems of draft-age young males stemmed from ignorance, low income, and limited access to care rather than deficits in scientific medical research. Fortunately, modern therapeutics helped modify these problems. Cardiorespiratory maneuvers to prevent and treat shock and better blood replacement techniques, including increase of the blood plasma supply, improved military medicine. In World War II less than 5 percent of wounded Americans died, about half the German mortality rate.

Application of the new drug therapies wrought a major transformation in U.S. hospitals, particularly in pediatric wards. Mortality from childhood infectious diseases and complications was drastically reduced in the 1940s. The overall death rate from pneumonia declined to 1 percent in 1944, compared to 24 percent before the advent of sulfa drugs. Mortality from meningitis was 38 percent in the World War I era and less than 5 percent by World War II. Children with congenital syphilis and atopic dermatitis were treated initially in pediatric dermatology. After penicillin made syphilis a rarity, more attention could be devoted to dermatology.

Before 1938, when the American Board of Plastic Surgery was founded, patients with harelips and cleft palates were sent to the Department of Otology, Rhinology, and Laryngology. World War II stimulated plastic and reconstructive surgery, much of which greatly enhanced the lives of children.[4]

In part because of the often poor physical condition of young male recruits, the war years brought preventive family health services to the forefront of the public welfare agenda. In Colorado the wives and children of men stationed in Denver, Colorado Springs, and elsewhere benefited from expansion of public health nursing and the Emergency Maternity and Infant Care Program (EMIC), inaugurated in 1943.[5] In 1945 paid medical care included more than 5,500 maternal and infant cases. The State Board of Health also continued child health conferences in permanent centers that also provided immunization clinics.

During the war virtually every business, public entity, and other organizations did their part to assist the war effort. This definitely included maintenance of a healthy, productive, civilian work force and its families. Children's Hospital provided in-service education programs for public health nurses in the state. The University of Colorado inaugurated a course for public health nurses in 1942, and during 1943 and 1944 nurses were brought to Children's for intensive training in the Sister Elizabeth Kenny method of using hot-wool packs and blankets in treating acute polio cases.[6] The state's Division of Crippled Children, a spinoff from the Social Security Act of 1935, served a large number of needy handicapped children. "Crippling" conditions subsumed any "remediable deformity or disease of the skeletal system . . . of a chronic nature," including harelip, cleft palate, and some remediable eye conditions such as congenital cataracts and traumatic cataracts. Children's expansion of physiotherapy and rehabilitation services reflected increasing awareness of the social, educational, and vocational services needed not only by wounded soldiers but also by the thousands of children handicapped by birth injury or crippling diseases.

In 1945 the Division of Crippled Children reported that many patients receiving excellent health care were "more handicapped from personality problems than from actual deformities. . . . Many young persons with handicapping physical conditions found it impossible to adapt themselves to the pressures and demands of the period."[7] Program officials urged more vocational rehabilitation services, plus additional convalescent and foster homes.

The State Board of Health praised numerous independent agencies that gave coordinated services to needy children, including Children's Hospital. The board noted that the Colorado Society for Crippled Children opened Sewall House in Denver to provide facilities for physical and occupational therapy for all kinds of crippling conditions. The National Foundation for Infantile Paralysis gave financial assistance and provided consultation services and treatment. The National Jewish Hospital opened a new ward for children with tubercular bone infections. Organizations such as the Rotary, Elks, and Lions Clubs, the Shriners, and the American Legion also supported these services.[8] At this time Children's Hospital also conformed to national trends in changing the label of physiotherapy to physical therapy.

The war years also marked intensified efforts to provide emergency neonatal care. In 1941 portable incubators were given to full-time health units, and public health nurses were assigned to rural areas. Most deaths among Colorado infants during 1944 were from premature birth (45.9 percent). Accordingly nurses were given special training in caring for these high-risk babies. They also demonstrated safe home care of premature infants to all public health care nurses in the state. Nursery supervisors in Denver hospitals produced a manual of safe nursing techniques in newborn nurseries.[9]

Because of a combination of explosive advances in new medical knowledge and advanced forms of treatment, rapid growth of Denver's population, large numbers of doctors returning from military service, and significant growth of state and federal funding, the postwar period saw many new clinics and scientific laboratories emerge at Children's Hospital.

The Infant Surgery Ward, established in 1948 under Dr. George Packard, Jr., and resident surgeon Dr. Levi Reynolds, was the result of rapid growth and increasing complexity in the diagnosis and treatment of congenital defects in infants. At first the new ward, served by special nurses, was only one small room with five bassinets; it filled to overflowing immediately. Burgeoning demand meant that it functioned as an intensive care unit, as patients could be held there only while in critical condition. Not until a decade later was the area expanded to hold thirty-two patients. The Infant Surgery Ward eventually evolved into the world-class Newborn Center.

Pediatric surgery had emerged fully with the founding of the American Board of Surgery in 1937. The work of Drs. William E. Ladd and Robert E. Gross at Boston Children's Hospital and publication of their textbook, *Abdominal Surgery in Infancy and Childhood,* in 1941 were landmark events in the evolution of full-fledged specialization in pediatric surgery. World War II military rank for doctors had depended on the amount of certified professional training. The high status attained by specialists, compared to general practitioners, encouraged many young doctors to take advantage of the GI Bill of Rights to continue their training after the war. Pediatric subspecialties were becoming more rooted in scientific research and education as well as in the new technology.[10]

Some of the new clinics at Children's Hospital emerged before the end of the war. In March 1943 the board approved conversion of the solarium into a modern laboratory, which opened in February of 1944. The old lab of three small rooms was converted to the X-ray Department, and new radiology equipment purchased by Mrs. Tammen before her death in 1942 was installed. The Roy P. Forbes Medical Library adjoined the new lab. Dr. Forbes, who died in 1943, was a favorite teacher of the residents and had served as medical staff president. He and Dr. W. Wiley Jones were founders of the clinical-pathological conferences.

The Blood Bank, established in 1943, stored blood for transfusion. Rh typing now gave hope to newborns with hemolytic disease caused by rhesus factor isoimmunization. Families and friends served as blood donors to avoid interfering with military needs in the Red Cross blood procurement program.[11] The new laboratory facilitated the first bone marrow aspiration biopsy in 1944. Dr. Harold D. Palmer maintained close personal relationships with East Coast "giants" in oncology-hematology, including Dr. Sidney Farber of Boston Children's Hospital. Palmer's career in oncologic therapy paralleled Farber's; thus he had knowledge of chemotherapy early in the history of pediatric oncology.

In 1946 the lab began diagnostic service for Rh-related erythroblastosis. On June 28, 1947, Dr. Edward L. Binkley carried out the first exchange transfusion at The Children's Hospital under the auspices of Dr. Harold Palmer and with the assistance of Dr. John Connell. Dr. Wayne Danielson was distressed at the wasted blood in these transfusions and began accumulating it for extensive analysis. His chemical data were the first to show a "profound degree of acidosis" present in the afflicted children before the transfusion. In the postwar period Danielson did extensive postgraduate

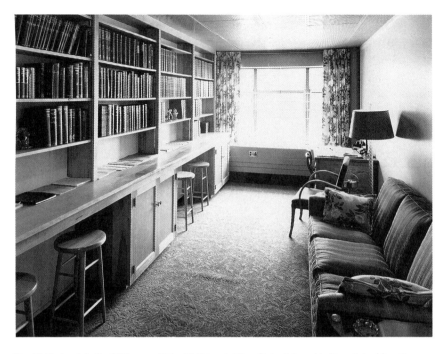

Roy P. Forbes Medical Library of The Children's Hospital, pictured in its original location on the fourth floor of the Agnes Reid Tammen building.

work at the world-renowned Mayo Clinic. In 1948 the first cardiac catheterization performed at Children's Hospital provided Danielson the opportunity to play a prominent role in analyzing the procedure's results.[12]

Thanks to the driving energy of Palmer, Danielson, and their colleagues, both equipment and procedures became increasingly sophisticated at Children's Hospital over the next few years. In August 1950 the first flame photometer was installed in the lab, probably one of the first used in a U.S. clinical laboratory. On April 12, 1951, a whole blood oximeter was used for the first time during cardiac catheterization.

In 1951 Dr. C. Richard Hawes was appointed fellow in pediatric cardiology, relieving Danielson of responsibility for supervising the Cardiac Laboratory. Danielson moved on to other new laboratory functions. At the beginning of 1953 Dr. Hawes helped establish use of an ear-piece oximeter used during surgery to monitor oxygen content of the blood. The first patient, referred by Dr. John Grow, was operated on for closure of a patent ductus arteriosus. The Van Slyke apparatus, plus equipment for respiratory gas analysis, was merged into a cardiopulmonary lab in the Department of Pathology, also in 1953. These instruments facilitated measurement of oxygen content of the blood.

At the end of 1953 Dr. Palmer was joined by Dr. Eugene Beatty as associate pathologist. After Palmer's resignation on July 1, 1955, Dr. Beatty became chief pathologist. In the late 1950s blueprints were drawn up for a definitive laboratory, and permanent space was occupied in 1961. The Women's Auxiliary (later renamed the Association of Volunteers) sponsored a carnival in the parking lot to raise funds for supporting equipment. Dr. Beatty continued in Palmer's tradition, serving as pathologist, hematologist, and oncologist until 1968.[13] He was joined for two years by Dr. William Reiquam, who was equally versatile. During this time the supervising physicians also expanded the cancer program at the hospital.

The Division of Clinical Chemistry emerged early in 1944 with the move to the remodeled solarium. Dr. Wayne Danielson had a fourfold mission. He first created a routine service to provide chemical analysis promptly to hospital physicians. The second goal was to incorporate new tests and instruments as they became available. For example, the spectrophotometer analyzed the vitamin content of blood, urine, and tissues. A third vital endeavor was reduction of necessary sample sizes. The development of microanalytic methods was obviously important in general pediatric medicine and particularly for premature and newborn infants. Finally the division developed a chemical research program. Postwar research projects included a study of new experimental techniques for increasing vitamin A absorption in patients with cystic fibrosis of the pancreas, and many others.

Miss Myrna Kempf developed the modern bacteriology lab for diagnostic and prognostic procedures. Routine studies included throat cultures for diagnosis and means of protecting children against other patients' contagious diseases. She also examined Rh incompatibility; these and other studies were reported in professional journals and meetings and in the new *Bulletin of The Children's Hospital*, first issued in January 1947 as a scientific quarterly.

In the latter stages of World War II a growing demand for treatment of children with neurologic damage evolved from the increasing survival of newborns with brain damage, the numbers of children recovering from

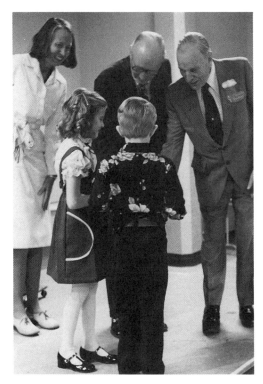

Lee Schlessman and Clarence Bartholic, members of
the Scottish Rite Foundation, are shown here accepting a gift from Carol Ehrlich, Ph.D., director of the
Department of Audiology and Speech Pathology, and
two children who have benefited from the generosity
of the foundation.

polio, and the growing load on the Physical and Occupational Therapy
Departments. The Cerebral Palsy Clinic, funded largely by a gift from the
Claude K. Boettcher family, opened on September 1, 1945. Mrs. Juliette M.
Gratke, formerly associated with the Children's Rehabilitation Institute
near Baltimore, was director. When she resigned in 1946, Dr. Edward
Binkley, the hospital's first research fellow, took her place.

On October 1, 1948, Speech and Hearing Clinics opened, under the
direction of Ruth Anderson and Marabeth Reid Terrell; forty-eight children
were enrolled by the end of the year. Their communication problems were
the result of cerebral palsy, deafness, aphasia, repaired cleft palates, or
stuttering and other conditions. In 1953 the hospital enlisted the gracious

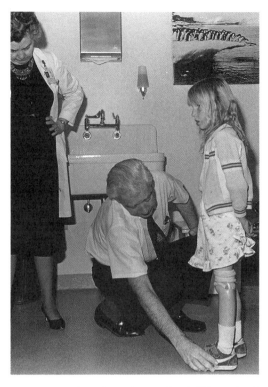

Dr. Jean McMahon, shown here with a child being fitted
for a prosthesis.

and vigorous assistance of the Scottish Rite Foundation, under the leadership of Mr. William G. Schweigert, to attack the problem of childhood
aphasia, thus providing funds to parents unable to pay for prolonged
therapy, for new equipment, and for an additional speech therapist.[14] Since
that time the Masonic Order and Children's Hospital have maintained a
partnership equally satisfying to both.

The Boettcher Evaluation Clinic, which later became the Developmental and Evaluation Clinic, opened in October 1956 and was staffed
part-time by Dr. Jean McMahon, who also directed the Outpatient Department. The Boettcher Clinic had one social worker, a psychologist, and a
secretary. Teams of private practitioners, including a pediatrician, a neu-
rologist, and an ophthalmologist, plus representatives from the Physical
Therapy, Occupational Therapy, and Speech Therapy Departments, met

once a month to examine four children. The clinic expanded to four teams in less than a year, but they could see only sixteen patients a month; the waiting list soon grew to several hundred children.[15]

The Pathology Department opened in 1943 and initially operated in only 322 square feet of space on the fifth floor. Despite cramped quarters and primitive equipment, the laboratory performed over 62,500 procedures in its first year. Meanwhile the staff optimistically drew sketches and outlined development of a new lab in the former convalescent ward, in disuse at the time because of wartime staff shortages.[16]

The opening of new laboratories, clinics, services, and whole new branches of medicine was an ongoing phenomenon at Children's Hospital in the 1940s and 1950s. In some departments experimentation and research were becoming increasingly important. Across the United States, research efforts in pediatric cardiology dated from the late nineteenth century, but little medical experimentation was done until the 1930s, when Dr. Helen Taussig's work helped merge embryology, physiology, and clinical skills. Her work sharpened diagnostic accuracy, leading to the first attempts at surgery. Although most of the pioneering advances in pediatric cardiology were achieved elsewhere, doctors at Children's Hospital kept abreast of the latest developments. During World War II, for example, Dr. George Packard, Jr., became the first doctor on the staff to perform patent ductus surgery.

Drs. Abe Ravin, Edgar Durbin, Carl Josephson, and Henry Bradford carried forward teaching, research, and clinical care in cardiology at Children's, dealing mostly with acquired disease. Dr. Ravin achieved a reputation as a superb teacher, in part for a unique system for teaching auscultation. He used controlled sound recordings in the classroom in order for students to become familiar with diagnostic murmurs and sounds before patient contact. He also led in developing cardiac catheterization techniques. Dr. Josephson was the first clinician at Children's to postulate intracranial arteriovenous fistula as a cause of heart failure in infancy and to elucidate the Bland-White-Garland syndrome. Dr. Durbin was warmly regarded as a "father figure" to rheumatic fever patients and children who had long stays at the hospital. Earl Petefish, later a successful barber in Littleton, long revered Durbin for enabling him to enjoy a productive adult life.

In the late 1940s and early 1950s Children's cardiologists conducted studies in the Radiology Department under Dr. R. Parker Allen, with considerable help from thoracic surgeon Dr. John Grow, assistant medical director Dr. John Connell, and clinical chemist Dr. Wayne Danielson. Danielson rapidly introduced new catheterization methods, using the microscholander technique for blood oxygen analysis. According to Dr. Hawes, "Many technicians wore out their patience, eyes and store of unprintable words as they strove into the nights trying to follow Dr. Danielson's strict techniques. . . . It was the firm conviction of all concerned that the tiny syringe-pipettes used in this method were surely works of the Devil himself." Despite such complaints, the clinicians obtained accurate data, leading in turn to more sophisticated diagnoses. Pathologist and medical director Harold Palmer recognized the central importance of the cardiac catheterization lab to hospital function and created a director's position, filled by Dr. Hawes.

Dr. Hawes credits Drs. Grow, Connell, and Allen with Children's "entry into the modern era of pediatric cardiology." Dr. Allen led the development of angiocardiography. He was "a master at pediatric plain film diagnosis" and introduced the Fairchild aerial camera into the lab. This was the predecessor of contemporary cineangiography equipment capable of providing rapid-sequence X-rays of injected contrast material passing through the heart. In one exercise using only standard, four-view cardiac series ordinary films, Dr. Allen correctly diagnosed 70 percent of the congenital defects cases without prior knowledge of historical or physical findings.

Dr. Grow was a key figure in the Cardiac Laboratory in the early 1950s. He came to Children's as a trained thoracic surgeon, picking up the patent ductus surgery where Dr. Packard left off. He did the first true "open-heart" procedure at the hospital: closure of an atrial septal defect. Early open-heart procedures were done under anesthesia and hypothermia, providing the surgeon only a few minutes to complete the internal repair. Dr. Grow pioneered this technique. Other ideas were tested, including an "immobile heart," "parabiosis," and use of early heart pumps.

The early cardiac teams, begun by Dr. Grow and his surgical nurse, Mrs. Kay Lundin, experienced failures and the subsequent wrenching deaths of some children. Drs. Charles DeMong and Arthur Prevedel joined the team, along with a second surgical nurse, Miss Rose Deneke. Dr. Hawes paid tribute to these pioneers: "The drain on all members of Children's early cardiac surgical team was tremendous, but they persisted and their work is now incorporated in the present cardio-pulmonary bypass techniques." Hawes modestly failed to mention his own enormous contribution. For years Hawes was the only pediatric cardiologist at Children's. From 1953 until the early 1970s he had full responsibility for operation of the lab and for patient care.[17]

Completion of an isolation unit for contagious diseases in 1942 evolved in response to the periodic polio epidemics that knew no socioeconomic bounds. The first patients were admitted to the new unit on January 29, 1943, the only facility in Denver to accept all forms of contagious disease. It boasted radiant air conditioning that warmed, filtered, and humidified the air in patients' rooms. Forty children could be cared for on its two floors; their most serious illnesses included polio, whooping cough, measles, diphtheria, severe chickenpox, dysentery from salmonella and shigella bacteria, meningitis, and hepatitis. There also were several cases of tuberculosis and viral encephalitis the first year.[18]

In 1942 the medical staff recognized the statewide crisis in a lack of services for polio victims and other crippled children. In response they made a precedent-breaking decision to admit children with acute polio so they could receive the new Sister Kenny treatment. This involved hot packing, followed by passive and active movement of the children's paralyzed extremities during the acute phase. Patients appeared to recover strength and range of motion more quickly than if physical therapy was delayed. A record 125 acute polio cases were admitted during 1943. The understaffed nursing personnel and six-member house staff, with Dr. Lula Lubchenco as chief resident, were inundated with the afflicted children. In 1944, although total hospital admissions increased 15 percent against the backdrop of staff and equipment shortages, acute-stage polio patients declined by more than half to fifty-seven.

The State Board of Health reported a total of only 604 cases between 1939 and 1944, and only 146 in 1945. But 1946 brought Colorado's worst polio epidemic to date, with 315 patients admitted to Children's Hospital alone through the summer and fall. Fortunately the hospital's response was dramatic and effective. Of those admitted to Children's in 1946, 192 were discharged as fully recovered. Several died, despite heroic, exhausting Sister Kenny treatments, which therapists and nurses provided around the clock, and an array of advanced technology. The National Foundation for Infantile Paralysis provided life-support equipment, additional nurses, physical therapists, and aides to relieve the desperately overworked staff. Local volunteers pitched in as well, many of them putting in the equivalent of a full work week. Some cases had highly dramatic results, with mixed news for their families. One pregnant woman was admitted with bulbar polio. She died in a Drinker respirator, but her infant was delivered alive and healthy.[19]

Children's Hospital did not battle the polio epidemic alone; other local hospitals contributed their services during the crisis. As the number of polio admissions steadily increased, convalescents were moved to Colorado General Hospital, where a converted student gymnasium served as a ward. As noncontagious bed space was filled at Children's, Denver General also took on some of the overflow. Early in June the State Board of Health banned T&A surgery, producing a backlog of these patients, who were not treated until after the epidemic subsided in November. Despite this closure of T&A beds, there were 7,906 total admissions to Children's, 1,366 more than in 1945. Another polio epidemic in 1951 brought 378 admissions with the disease, out of a total of 13,000 admissions during the hospital's busiest year yet.

The annual report for 1952 documented the increasing survival rate in polio cases with more new treatments. Three hundred new polio patients were admitted, with the bulbar type involving more treatment of neck, throat, face, shoulder, and arm dysfunction. Thus there was an increasing need for speech therapy, plus treatments for many other muscle groups. In 1952, 274 were admitted, only forty-seven in 1953, and eighty-nine two years later. Fortunately the new Salk vaccine was introduced, and polio cases decreased dramatically. Dr. Hawes recalled the exciting announcement of Dr. Jonas Salk's breakthrough. Several hundred physicians and other health care experts were invited to the Paramount Theater in downtown Denver, where the welcome news was officially delivered amidst tremendous fanfare. The victory over the dreaded affliction was swift and almost totally complete. In 1955 only one polio victim receiving Salk vaccine had residual paralysis. With the great decrease in polio patients, the Isolation Unit managed to treat a much broader range of serious illnesses.[20]

In fact, the new techniques for treating hospital patients at Children's and other hospitals had been evolving for many years. One historian describes the modern United States hospital of the late 1930s as a "marvel of engineering," run by a "technological bureaucracy." Like hundreds of other hospitals across the country, Children's modernized with state-of-the-art air-control systems, refrigeration, centralized culinary units, and central supply rooms.[21] Modern hospitals provided stage sets of biotechnical drama for daily life-and-death scenes. These and other futuristic design applications in the ward rooms, corridors, and reception areas symbolized the vital energy exuded by the army of health care professionals.

With the end of World War II many young doctors returned home, eager to resume interrupted medical careers and make up for lost time. One promising avenue for ambitious doctors and staff members was a distinct departure from full-time practice of applied medicine: research and the advancement of medical knowledge. This new development, with encouragement from Drs. Harold Palmer and George Packard, Jr., inspired large monthly attendance of from fifty to 100 staff members at surgical section meetings.

Annual summer clinics, begun in 1946, also publicized advanced work in pediatric surgery at Children's, highlighting its rapidly evolving image as a unique regional specialty hospital. These three-day meetings featured presentations by eminent pediatricians, surgeons, pathologists, radiologists, and other experts from around the country. The summer clinics regularly attracted 200 or more professionals, many from other towns in Colorado, Wyoming, and western Kansas and Nebraska. On February 7, 1946, Children's hosted the first Mid-Winter Postgraduate Clinic of the Colorado State Medical Society. Drs. W. Wiley Jones and Harold Palmer continued bimonthly clinical-pathologic conferences, with cases reported in the *Bulletin*. The Denver County Medical Society also chose the hospital for its October 1946 meeting.[22]

In the postwar period major changes in U.S. medical practice were clearly in the wind. Eagerly taking up the scepter of medical research from fallen research establishments in war-devastated European nations, U.S. medical schools stressed training of investigators as well as practitioners.[23] Research increasingly brought prestige plus both private and government-funded grants. Dr. Blaise Favara, an active scholar, claimed that Children's entrance into the realm of research "really begins with Dr. Harold Palmer's acceptance of the position of Pathologist and Medical Director of the Hospital in 1942." Palmer became a "vitalizing force in the development of the laboratory services and in all aspects of the medical education program." In his report as retiring medical staff president, Dr. Atha Thomas called the appointment of Dr. Palmer "the most important and successful accomplishment of the year."[24]

Palmer stated three objectives for his tenure, which lasted until 1955: continuing the tradition of excellence in laboratory medicine; reorganizing the residency training program; and a commitment to research and education vital to progress in pediatrics. He recruited Miss Myrna Kempf as bacteriologist and Dr. Wayne Danielson as clinical chemist, and they commenced an aggressive expansion program. The laboratories were divided into bacteriology, chemistry, hematology, and pathology.

In a speech to the medical staff in 1952, retiring president Dr. Max Ginsburg acknowledged a shift in the hospital's mission that had been in motion for several years:

> Children's Hospital should not merely be a place where children get good treatment and services for their illness. Many of the general hospitals do that and if we are to exist and grow we must offer something more. We must lead in the newer forms of therapy, which only a specialized hospital can offer. To interest the men of the highest caliber to bring their patients here as well as to obtain well qualified residents, this institution should be a source of intellectual stimulation.[25]

The large patient load and excellent facilities gave Children's the potential to become a premier clinical research institution. A handful of staff doctors had already made scholarly contributions. Despite severe wartime restrictions Drs. Lula Lubchenco and Wayne Danielson studied nutritional disorders under a Mead Johnson Laboratories grant. They presented a paper on fat metabolism and absorption at a meeting of the American Society of Clinical Pathologists; it was published in the *Journal of Clinical Pathology*. Other studies brought national attention to Children's Hospital.[26]

In 1953 The Children's Hospital Research Foundation was established but without immediate funding for projects. The most dramatic medical development of 1953 was the performance of cardiac surgery under hypothermia. A twenty-two-month-old infant had one of the first operations of its kind in the region. The baby was anesthetized, then immersed in ice cubes and cooled to 75 degrees Fahrenheit; then the valvular stenosis was corrected. Others were operated on in succeeding months, including a four-month-old baby with a severe Tetralogy of Fallot. He weighed only five pounds, six ounces but showed marked improvement in oxygenation following his recovery.

Neurosurgery at Children's Hospital reflected the increasing skill and training needed to stay abreast of rapid technical advances in surgery

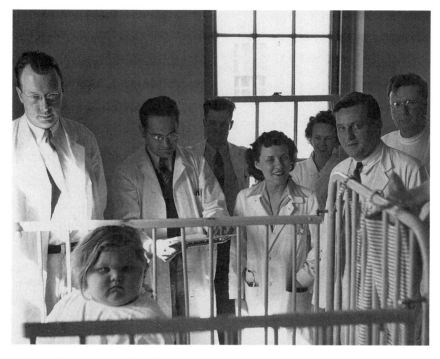

Dr. Harry Gordon (second from left), first full-time professor of pediatrics at the University of Colorado Medical Center, making rounds with residents Drs. Marvin Becker, Lameta Dahl, Lula Lubchenco, and Brian Moynihan in 1946. (Two men, the man behind Gordon and the man behind Moynihan, are unidentified.)

nationwide. The career profile of one notable doctor at Children's is representative. Dr. William R. Lipscomb finished training at the Mayo Clinic in neurosurgery in 1938. When he returned to Denver, Dr. George Packard, Jr., warned him that he faced severe competition in his chosen field. Suddenly, however, Lipscomb's reputation rose. Pediatrician Roderick J. McDonald asked him to examine a young boy who was incoordinate and had crossed eyes and severe headaches. Dr. Lipscomb diagnosed a cerebellar tumor and cyst. The anesthetist used a new method of intratracheal anesthesia, and Dr. Lipscomb performed a suboccipital craniotomy, drained a large cyst, and removed the tumor. Convalescence went well, and the child became coordinate.

He had similar success with a five-year-old girl who had a vascular lesion of the right cerebrum. Following a craniotomy at Johns Hopkins

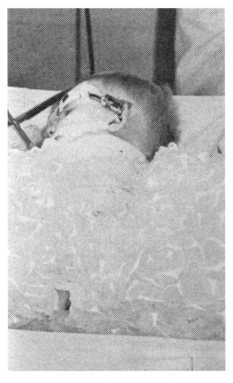

Patient seen immersed in ice cubes during one of
first open-heart surgeries of its kind in the region,
introduced and pioneered by Dr. John B. Grow,
Sr.

Hospital, she returned to Denver. Unfortunately her blood pressure remained high and she had albuminuria; she was readmitted to Children's
Hospital for renal studies. Exploratory surgery revealed an aneurysm
involving the pedicle of the kidney. The scene in the operating room was
one of high drama. An emergency decision to remove the kidney was
concurred in by her father, an Episcopal priest. He stood in the corner of
the room and urged the physician to take it out, while the medical team
debated. Despite one technician's concern that the abnormal pathology
surely involved the other kidney and would cause her death, Lipscomb
saved the young patient and she thrived. He continued his exacting surgical
practice in Denver from 1939 to 1942, when he joined the armed forces.[27]

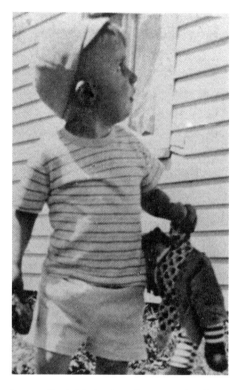

Same patient able to play after recovering from
the surgery and hypothermia technique.

After his return from service, Lipscomb had the opportunity to treat
or examine most known types of pathological conditions of the brain and
spinal cord. Children's provided him an excellent workshop and supporting colleagues. According to Lipscomb he and Dr. Palmer's residents were
assisted by the "best pediatric nursing care in any Denver hospital."

Lipscomb was appointed to the executive committee of the medical
staff by Dr. Ralph Verploeg in 1947. Lipscomb urged acquisition of an
electroencephalograph because many patients admitted to Children's with
convulsive disorders had to be taken elsewhere for the EEG. The board
granted his request. He also urged use of the Spitz-Holter valve for hydro-
cephalus in infants, developed by a neurosurgeon at Philadelphia's Children's Hospital.

Gradually, almost imperceptibly, Children's Hospital broadened its mission. For decades the institution had attracted reputable practitioners whose professional lives revolved around hands-on healing — direct contact with patients. A few prominent doctors were interested in advancing medical knowledge through research, but most experienced short tenure at Children's, then moved on. In the 1950s, however, a culture of theoretical as well as applied research gradually emerged from the labs and discussions in the doctors' and surgeons' lounges.

In 1956 medical director John R. Connell left little doubt that research was becoming an integral, respected responsibility of many doctors at Children's: "no longer does it suffice for Children's Hospital to provide its particular standard of superior patient care." Echoing Ginsburg's words of four years earlier, Connell acknowledged "a professional and moral obligation to foster the advancement of medical science as it particularly applies to prevention, diagnosis, and treatment of diseases of infancy and childhood." The director singled out a rising star, Dr. Hawes, who, "with members of the Staff . . . developed a coronary artery perfusion technique, using siliconed apparatus and arterialized venous blood."[28]

Within a few years important scholarly work by Children's doctors was quite common; only particularly noteworthy published articles, papers, and other contributions were mentioned in the hospital's publicity reports. By the end of the 1950s the hospital emerged as a center for a handful of specialized services, including cardiac surgery and critical care for newborns. Children's was not yet a leader at the national level, but it had clearly developed a leading regional position in specialized care of children.

Despite increased attention to research and specialization, the hospital's focus remained very much on the immediate, practical task of making children well. Although crowding and confusion occasionally obscured the larger purpose of doctors and staff, for the most part young patients quickly sensed that they were in very capable hands. Doctors, nurses, and volunteers were particularly adept at persuading children to deal realistically with their own illnesses, yet to perceive their situations in the best possible light. One volunteer recalled helping move a young patient who had been in an iron lung for several months to another room. Another child in apparent distress was wheeled past her. When told the patient's diagnosis, she blurted out, "Boy, I'm glad I'm not a tonsil kid."[29]

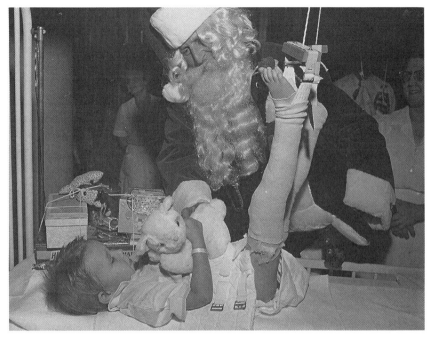

For years Santa Claus (Mel Schlesinger) visited hospitalized children bringing gifts and the spirit of Christmas. Photo from the *Denver Post*.

Parents of former patients testified repeatedly concerning the warmth and compassion of all who served their children. One woman recalled a Christmas in the late 1940s when her grandson was alone at Children's except for occasional visits by his father, who lived far away. The little boy was thrilled with a Christmas visit by Santa: "He did not think Santa would find him there in the hospital. Santa brought him two nice presents [which] . . . were right down his alley." Other parents, proud but often poor, eloquently expressed their gratitude when large portions of their children's bills were cancelled or covered by the Tammen Fund. In 1957 Richard Gottardi's daughter Lisa required an operation for a cleft palate. The family was in dire financial straits, and the Tammen Fund came to the rescue. The father expressed his gratitude for "kind deeds such as yours [which] appear as a gentle and pacifying breeze in the driving storms of a chaotic life." Many recipients of relief from burdensome debts expressed a strong desire

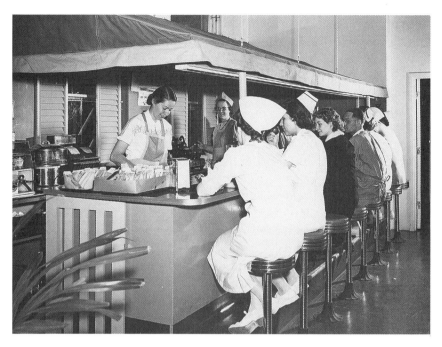

Babs Humphreys preparing food in the snack bar, paid for and staffed by the Junior League of Denver. At the end of two years the operations were turned over to the Auxiliary of the hospital.

to repay money into the fund when circumstances permitted. Some actually did so. In the summer of 1956 the Helmer Hendricksons' son Johnny required an operation. When he left the hospital, the balance due was $332. Nine months later Mrs. Hendrickson proudly paid in full. Some who could not pay cash donated toys for Christmas gifts or blood for others in need.[30] More than any spectacular operation or brilliant research paper, the generosity of hospital benefactors and the gentleness and kindness of doctors, nurses, staff, and volunteers remained the foundation stones of Children's Hospital's well-deserved regional reputation.

As medical care became increasingly technical and specialized, hospital administrators made a concerted effort to keep the atmosphere humane, informal, and relaxed — in short, child-centered. Volunteerism retained a high profile in day-to-day life in the hospital. Children could not leave the hospital without having some contact with volunteers, most of them women. The Women's Auxiliary, formally organized in 1948, quickly grew to more than 300 members. One monthly summary from 1952 of hours volunteered reported: office work, 283 hours; transportation for patients, 195; hostess functions, 132; dressing and caring for children, 98; helping nurses feed babies and handicapped patients, 91; and 68 hours helping admit and examine patients. The Junior League of Denver paid for and staffed a snack bar at Children's Hospital, which opened in 1950, as well as a gift shop. For two years the Junior League divided profits from the snack bar and gift shop with the hospital. In 1952 the league turned these projects over to the Auxiliary. Finally, the women volunteers organized and managed numerous additional fund-raisers: luncheons, teas, fashion shows, designers' show-home tours, and other forms of entertainment.[31] In many respects the nature of the volunteers' commitments changed little in forty years.

Agnes Tammen was undoubtedly the most visible philanthropist up to her death in 1942. She supplied Children's Hospital with the latest equipment, but she and hundreds of her less well-known peers also worked hard to keep the environment from being stark and impersonal. Interior designers emphasized color patterns of soft greens and grays typical in hospitals of the era. The *Denver Post* praised the "democracy" of the environment; no distinction was made between paying and charity patients. "Viewed as a civic asset, Children's hospital is regarded as the rarest crown jewel of [the] community," the paper stated. Renowned outsiders also shared that view. During a personal visit Sister Elizabeth Kenny, a pioneer in polio treatment, was remembered for the warmth of her voice in murmuring how beautiful Children's environment was. The Reverend John T. Smith, bishop of the Episcopal diocese of London, proffered his blessing: "Wonderful . . . God's word made manifest."[32]

In the eyes of young patients many doctors and staff members seemed almost like saints. One example was Mr. Gosta Valdemar, who took over as director of the Physiotherapy Department after Director Witham's abrupt departure. Young Bill Shafer, a polio victim, never forgot how "Gus" Valdemar transformed his life. When admitted, the young patient was in pitiful condition, his heels drawn up to his thighs, his thighs to his chest. He was placed in traction to straighten his legs, and he remained in a dreaded cast for six months. His parents were advised that he would not live past thirty-five and that his heart could not stand the strain of ever leaving his bed.

Bill Shafer proved the "experts" wrong. Fifty years later he recalled the beginning of his fight to lead a normal life. "One morning this big blond giant came to my hospital bed and said, 'Hi, I'm Gus, and I understand you want to walk.'" Valdemar had been Sweden's "most perfectly developed man." Becoming interested in polio and physical therapy, he came to the United States where there were more postpolio patients and handicapped persons to work with.

One of Gus's strategies was to challenge his young charges. After a few days of therapy Gus told Shafer that he should be able to get up and walk: "Frankly I don't believe you have the guts to do it because you're spoiled and a cry-baby, and you'll have to change your entire attitude. Do you think you're man enough to do it?" Young Bill rose to the challenge, exercising for hours each day and attending school during his breaks from physical therapy. Painfully he managed to walk a few more inches each day.

When Gus left the hospital, however, for several weeks' training in Sister Kenny's treatment at President Roosevelt's famous retreat in Warm Springs, Georgia, Bill suffered a relapse. During Gus's absence physicians had put Shafer back into a full-body cast after a fall broke his arm. Shafer soon despaired of ever getting out of his wheelchair. Sizing up his young charge's ennui, Gus showed no pity when he returned. Instead he cut him out of his body cast immediately and recommended vigorous training. Gus worked hard on Bill's stride and the art of falling by kicking out his crutch unexpectedly, so that his protective reflexes came into play instinctively.

Valdemar also won over his patients by good-natured defiance of some of the "authorities." He was a pal to the handicapped children, occasionally outwitting the night supervisor, whom Bill called "Old Pussyfoot" with crepe-soled shoes. One night she came in after Gus had smuggled about fifty hamburgers into the ward. "Swish-swish" came the shoes, as Old Pussyfoot's flashlight beamed into the party. She demanded to know what was going on and disdainfully said she smelled onions. Levity prevailed, and the hamburger parties became a weekly ritual. The conspirators began ordering extras for the ward nurses, and even for Old Pussyfoot. When Bill left the hospital for good, Gus told him that together they had "rewritten the book on rehabilitation." Gus continued to be a part of Bill's family life, and over the years Bill married, fathered four sons, supported his family, and became a grandfather.[33]

Meanwhile, serious business and crises continued during the immediate postwar years, interspersed with some amusing incidents. Dr. Seymour Wheelock survived his childhood tonsillectomy, became a pediatrician, and began his residency at Children's in 1946. Pediatricians at this time battled infectious diseases such as strep throat, pneumonia, rheumatic fever, diphtheria, polio, and tuberculosis. Antibiotics were still in short supply; Dr. Wheelock recalled that as many as a third of the 300 to 400 pneumonia patients died in 1946. Other wartime crises affected the patients at Children's. One night a crash at Lowry Air Force Base knocked out the electricity. At first the residents considered the blackout amusing, until they remembered eight patients on respirators. They bolted up the steps two at a time and spent the rest of the night manually operating the respirators.

An amusing incident involved frivolous use of the new radiology equipment. One night when reading X-ray films, Dr. Verploeg had nonchalantly slipped one into the stack; a fellow doctor gasped with disbelief at seeing five skeletons in one pregnant body. The "patient" was one of Dr. Verploeg's pregnant, prize red setters![34]

These years were marked by healthy growth and expanding opportunities for doctors and high-level support staff. For the rest of the hospital workers, future prospects probably did not appear so bright. Nationwide, blue-collar militancy was increasing. Yet the workers at Children's Hospital chose to exclude themselves from union organizing, which mushroomed after 1935 with the help of federal legislation under the Industrial Labor Relations Act and the formation of industrial unions in the CIO under John L. Lewis. Hospital culture, still based on hierarchical arrangements and paternalism symbolized in doctor-patient, doctor-nurse, and nurse-patient relationships, did not nurture worker democracy. Nevertheless at many hospitals, including Children's, staff personnel were becoming restive. The Witham incident had signified a degree of alienation among some workers, particularly women. Physiotherapy was a high-profile physical occupation, involving many female therapists working in close physical contact with male patients — and doctors. The potential for misunderstandings and conflict was high, probably exacerbated by the likelihood that some female therapists felt thwarted in their efforts to become doctors.

"Troublemakers" of either gender gained little support in hospital power structures nationwide. But the spreading bureaucracies gradually challenged traditional physician authority by sheer strength of numbers.

From 1936 to 1942 the number of lab technicians almost doubled; X-ray technicians and pharmacists increased by over two-thirds, with smaller but important increases in dietitians and physical therapists. Not only did nonmedical female professionals challenge the dominance and autonomy of male doctors, but so did a bevy of college-educated administrators, with their new ideas about organization and managerial efficiency.

Whatever internal tensions may have emerged, the postwar hospital staff grew in all categories. Medical men returned from military service. Residents who trained in rapidly expanding postwar specialty programs at various local hospitals also found the region desirable and many stayed. There were thirty men on the active surgical staff. Dr. George Packard, Jr., a nationally renowned pediatric surgeon, handled all "difficult" cases and maintained a practice for adults as well as children. Dr. David R. Akers was the first Denver surgeon to confine his work entirely to infants and children, beginning in 1953. He later was joined in his specialty by Drs. William C. Bailey, John D. Burrington, Eli Wayne, George Peters, Jack Chang, and others.[35]

Physicians were suddenly abundant. Staff returning from military service had top priority for appointments, leaving very few positions available for newcomers. There was a major bed shortage, and with the development of increasingly sophisticated and labor-intensive procedures, the house staff was insufficient to handle the growing patient load and faster daily pace at Children's Hospital. These factors led to persistent pressure for further expansion of the hospital, but this would not occur until the late 1950s.

With prosperity and rapid population growth in the metropolitan region in the postwar decade, demand for medical care could only increase. The University of Colorado Medical School thrived in this environment, and its association with Children's deepened. Children's was approved for residency training by the American Board of Surgery in 1946, and residents from the University of Colorado provided service in ever-increasing numbers.[36]

In 1949 two residents in orthopaedics, one in surgery, two in pathology, and seven in pediatrics completed training. Programs were fully accredited, with high percentages of graduates succeeding in examinations for specialty board certification. Most remained to practice in the Rocky Mountain and Great Plains regions, in order to have continued access to experienced Children's Hospital staff, some with national reputations. Dr.

Palmer was elected to the board of governors of the American College of Pathologists and became associate editor of the society's journal. Dr. John Connell became a member of the American Academy of Pediatrics Committee on Hospital Care of Children, continuing for five years. These men, along with their junior colleagues, had the benefit of overseeing a thousand new patients a month and working with serious medical problems unique to children.[37] Such opportunities helped attract a number of young and gifted doctors, including Dr. C. Richard Hawes who came as a resident. Hawes also had "family ties" to the hospital, being related to Dr. John Amesse, Jr. Dr. Hawes recalled living in the same row of townhouses occupied by residents for a generation. Although residents, unlike nurses, did not have curfew, in some ways they were still regarded as adolescents, having to sneak extra food from the kitchen or to circumvent particularly mid-Victorian hospital rules when Oca Cushman was not looking.[38]

Even Mrs. Cushman, an institution within an institution, could not go on forever. She announced her retirement in February 1955, ending forty-five years of continuous service. The medical staff and 700 friends and associates celebrated her career and bid her an affectionate farewell. During her long reign over the domestic needs and comforts of patients and staff, she represented both the old and the new and Children's balance between traditional caregiving and innovative therapeutics and procedures.

Medicine was dominated by males, and Oca was comfortable with this. In many ways the Victorian lady, she insisted on propriety in behavior of all her charges but tended to be much harder on women. She inspected nurses' quarters with white gloves, looking for hidden dirt. According to Dr. Jean McMahon, romances were discouraged among the support staff. McMahon also believed that Oca was confounded by overly ambitious women: "When I became an intern [in 1940] Mrs. Cushman didn't know what to do with me since I was a woman, so she put me in the nurse's dorm and gave me a curfew of 10 P.M."[39] Ironically it was not until 1955, the same year Mrs. Cushman announced her retirement, that a female physician was chosen president of the medical staff. The precedent-breaking pediatrician was Dr. Mariana Gardner, a popular and energetic physician who was active in the affairs of Children's Hospital in her private practice until her death in 1962.

The 1950s marked the departure of other "living monuments" at the hospital. Dr. Palmer, who had been instrumental in modernizing the hospital's mission to emphasize medical education and research, retired in

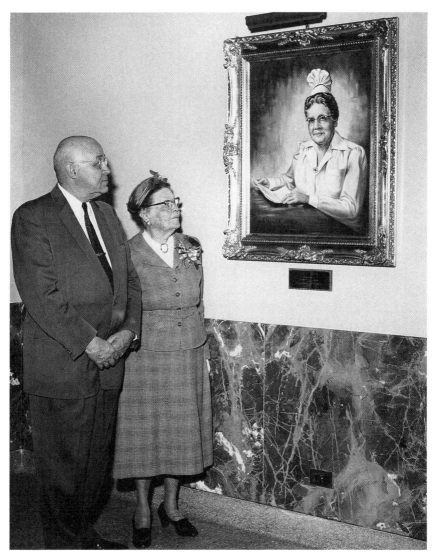

DeMoss Taliaferro, director of the hospital, with Mrs. Oca Cushman at the time of her retirement after forty-five years.

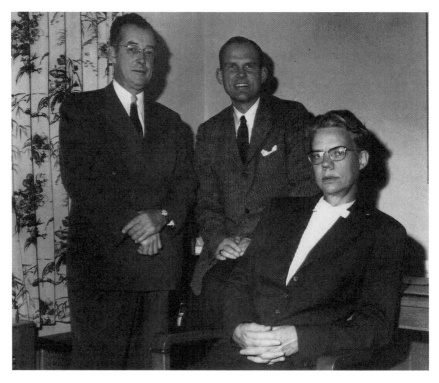

Dr. Mariana Gardner, first and only woman president of the medical staff, shown here with Drs. Edwin T. Williams and Seymour E. Wheelock, partners with Dr. Gardner in private practice.

June 1955 and returned to Illinois. In 1958 hospital director DeMoss Taliaferro also retired after twenty-one years on the job. Taliaferro and Cushman were symbols of an older managerial style: highly personalized as opposed to bureaucratic or scientific. Later generations of managers relied increasingly on bureaucratic policy, feasibility studies, statistics, and computerized printouts in decision making. Taliaferro and Cushman generally relied on direct, one-to-one conversations, handwritten memos, personal observation, long experience, and instincts.

During and after the war Children's Hospital emerged as a full-blown pediatric and orthopaedic hospital with national stature. New drugs and the seemingly miraculous conquest of hitherto fatal infectious diseases reinforced the image of the doctor as a "figure of authority," almost god-like.[40] Fortunately many doctors had the good sense not to take themselves too seriously. Dr. L. Joseph Butterfield worked with singular passion to gain for the Newborn Center a national reputation. When he arrived as a resident in 1956, he immediately noticed a pecking order, and in his early years Butterfield showed proper deference to the medical hierarchy. He was privately amused when one particularly pompous, attending physician gestured toward a patient's chart, demanding to know of Alice Alcott, R.N., "What does this number indicate?" Alcott responded matter-of-factly: "That's the date, doctor." Some doctors insisted on being treated like visiting royalty. Another physician observed that "protocol was rigid in those days." Both nurses and residents stood when a doctor entered the ward, often addressing him with military precision: "Yes, Doctor" or "No, Doctor."[41]

In private, younger residents were not always complimentary toward superiors. Many detested tonsil-ward duty. One raconteur recalled: "Tonsils were removed almost automatically when a child was four and often the surgeons would not spend enough time cauterizing the wound. So we residents spent hours trying to stop the bleeding. It was a nightmare." For the most part, however, patients and staff memories of doctors' treatments and, equally important, their commitment and compassion were highly laudatory.[42]

Some staff muttered softly about poor treatment of nurses by doctors, but that alone could not explain the chronic shortage in the profession. By mid-century, hospitals nationwide felt the pinch. Wage scales and working conditions discouraged many potential nurses. The number of graduate staff nurses dropped precipitously. This was partly because of higher pay, more status, and increasing opportunities in competing skilled professional and white-collar jobs. Although millions of women had been pressured to abandon fulfilling jobs after World War II, largely in deference to returning male veterans, the unprecedented prosperity of the 1950s created vast new professional opportunities. Fewer women were willing to endure the long hours and regimented working conditions that were the hallmark of nursing school.[43]

In an employee's marketplace hospitals competed vigorously to attract and retain first-rate skilled nurses. In 1952 Children's awarded bonuses to nurses serving a full year and made other concessions, but still it suffered a net loss of nurses. In 1953 the directors decided to close the basic nursing school. At the time, it was one of only two such schools in the nation directly connected to a hospital. Too often Children's could not induce its own graduates to return after they took specialized training elsewhere. In 1954 admissions were closed; the last entering class graduated in 1956. This trend was typical. In California, for example, both the Children's Hospital of San Francisco and Kaiser Permanente closed nursing training facilities at the same time.[44]

Unfortunately some of the strategies supervisors used to cover nurse shortages further antagonized those remaining. They recruited part-time professionals and student nurses, who were paid by the hour. The head nurse streamlined procedures to shift nurses from one specialty to another in emergencies, and she delegated more of her clerical duties to subordinates so she could keep a closer eye on nurses' performance. Doctors fretted because they feared that nurses assigned to them might be insufficiently prepared to handle emergencies. Sensitive nurses perceived a lessening of professional respect by some physicians, and some viewed the changes as a thinly disguised speedup. One short-term solution was that volunteers in the auxiliary took over some of the nurses' less critical tasks.[45] Still, stress increased in every facet of the job.

Growth figures alone helped explain the enormous pressure on the staff during the 1940s and 1950s. In 1940 there were 3,846 admissions, of whom 2,069 were either free or only part-pay. During the war years charity cases dropped, in part because the economic boom meant fewer poor families. A year after the war's outbreak, almost 60 percent of patients paid their entire bills.[46] Between 1942 and 1952 admissions jumped from 5,549 to 13,663. In 1954 the numbers dropped markedly, to 10,103, partly because of dramatic increases in outpatient treatment.

The course of many diseases was favorably altered by new drugs, and more children could be handled on an outpatient basis. In 1948 the hospital provided 13,191 outpatient treatments: physical therapy accounted for 4,555; occupational therapy, 2,323; and X-ray services, 2,110. In a decade outpatient services almost tripled. By 1957 some 36,091 visits were recorded, as Children's emerged as a regional leader in physical and occupational therapy. In 1948 the speech clinic provided 684 treatments; just six years later the number exceeded 10,000. Thanks to generous support from the Boettcher Foundation and the Scottish Rite Foundation, the Speech Clinic became justifiably renowned. Equally important, therapists at Children's regularly demonstrated new experimental techniques for the benefit of other professionals in the region.[47] Such outreach portended the hospital's spreading regional influence in the second half of the century.

Despite occasional dips in admissions, the general trend was upward. The hospital creaked and groaned with the relentlessly expanding patient load. Chief of surgery George Packard, Jr., reported that the operating suite was in a "particularly precarious status." From 1940 to 1952 surgery on children under six years of age had nearly trebled. Yet operating facilities were largely unchanged since 1917 when Children's had only sixty-five beds. The greatest space needs were for operating rooms, an X-ray department, laboratories, and more room for the care of infants and small children. The board began developing a building program to meet these needs.[48]

Increasing emphasis on outpatient treatment was in part a response to escalating costs for inpatient treatment and the fact that private insurers simply were not protecting enough Americans. This was true nationwide and at Children's. An admissions officer reported in 1939 that just over half of the parents bringing children to the hospital had any private coverage, and some policies had benefit ceilings as low as $50.[49] More parents had automobiles than health insurance. Senator Robert A. Wagner (D-NY) and a handful of liberal colleagues in Congress had passionately promoted national health insurance since the mid-1930s, but the AMA and private insurance companies had effectively countered their efforts.

For most of the first half of the twentieth century medical costs were modest, and these issues did not constitute a crisis. By the late 1940s the situation was changing, and private insurers were clearly not meeting the needs of the "bottom half" of the nation's consumers. Other factors contributed to the health care dilemma, making it more complex and frustrating. Hospital director DeMoss Taliaferro and Blue Cross negotiated several contracts establishing fixed fees for most services. Although contracts were apparently worked out in good faith, rampant inflation made them obsolete almost before the ink dried. In 1949 Taliaferro reported the hospital's net loss was "about equal to our Blue Cross losses." After mid-century, inflation temporarily abated, and hospital administrators became more skilled in contract negotiations with insurers. Health plans gradually improved by the end of the 1950s; roughly 70 percent of patients' families were privately insured. Nevertheless hospital administrators and board members had not yet developed a sophisticated perception of financial realities in health care. For years the Tammen Trust had provided a buffer against

many of the uncompromising facts in the vigorous competition for philanthropic support. Only at the last minute was the task of "seeking annual,
continuing grants from Foundations and individuals" added to the board's
agenda for 1957.

Beset by unprecedented challenges in the postwar years, the board
improvised, worked long hours, and doggedly did its best. By the early
1950s, however, one challenge demanded long-term planning: space needs.
In 1940 Dr. George Packard, Jr., had recommended expansion of surgical
rooms and other facilities. The board responded favorably, but wartime
exigencies prevented action. Since then surgery had multiplied several-
fold, yet no expansion occurred. Ancillary services were, if anything, even
more cramped, and many areas of the hospital had a run-down, even
dreary look.[50]

In 1952 the board again authorized expansion, and over the next year
and a half planning progressed rapidly. Fund-raising was the most critical
task, with all money expected to come from private sources. As they had
in 1916, the board hired a private firm. This time Will, Folsom and Smith
of New York helped raise $1.25 million. As planning progressed, respon-
sible officials soon raised their budget to $2.4 million, adding several
additional offices. Detailed plans were submitted to doctors, nurses, and
administrators for suggestions; the process was remarkably democratic.

What may have consumed the least time was choosing a name for the
new wing. The board voted to name it after Oca Cushman, who had not
yet announced her retirement. The new wing, constructed to the north
between 1954 and 1957, was a three-story addition containing nearly 73,000
square feet of space. Air-conditioned throughout, it housed four major and
four minor surgery rooms, a recovery room, four cast and two fracture
rooms, two emergency rooms, and six examining rooms. Reflecting the
concerns of the broad array of medical professionals who influenced the
planning of the new facility, it also included space for medical education,
diagnosis of diseases, doctors' and surgeons' lounges, offices and conference rooms, ward space for nearly 100 bassinets and cribs, a premature
nursery, and a children's playroom. In addition to two dining rooms, a
cafeteria, and modern kitchen services, the new wing also contained storage space, machine rooms, and numerous service and reception areas for
the public. The entire wing was built and equipped within the revised
budget.[51]

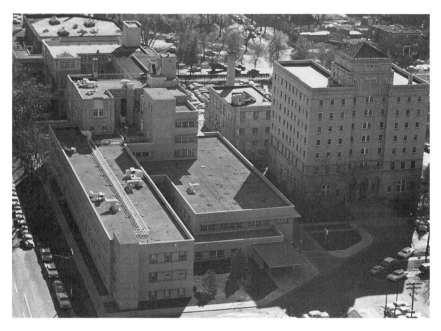

In October 1965 the Oca Cushman Wing, a three-story addition shown in the foreground and bordered by Downing Street and Nineteenth Avenue, opened; it was dedicated to the woman who gave a lifetime of love and devotion to the children of Denver. Photo taken from a helicopter on November 7, 1962, by Yugi Oishi, medical photographer at Children's.

The 1940s and 1950s brought unprecedented problems and challenges to leaders at Children's. Yet given the national crisis in virtually all phases of health care delivery in the early 1990s, the challenges of these earlier years appear almost minuscule, even quaint. For example, up to this point the hospital had operated almost entirely free of government support or regulation; the "ma and pa" administrative procedures employed in earlier years appear almost ridiculously simplistic today. Physicians and hospital administrators had less reason to worry about malpractice suits. Medical ethics committees were unknown, but doctors of the 1940s and 1950s experienced challenges equally serious in learning about new generations of antibiotics and changing long-held assumptions concerning dozens of procedures. By the end of the 1950s an aura of change was ever-present, and it would intensify dramatically in the years just ahead.

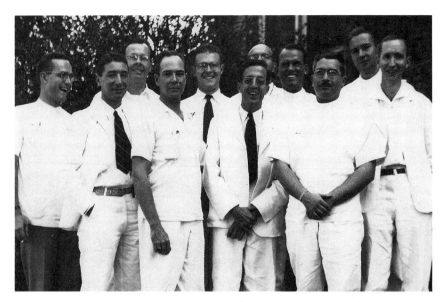

Residents 1946–1947: (front row) Drs. John Connell, David Akers, William Robb, Joseph Goran, and James Watson; (back row) Drs. Prather Ashe, Marvin Becker, Bedford Berry, Charles Hranac, Seymour E. Wheelock, and Murray Gibbons.

Notes

1. DeMoss Taliaferro, in *Thirtieth Annual Report* (1940), Historical Number for Thirtieth Anniversary, CHD Collection.

2. Rosemary Stevens, *In Sickness and in Wealth: American Hospitals in the Twentieth Century* (New York: Basic Books, Inc., 1989), 177–178; quotation in Stevens, 394, n.19, from Morris F. Collin, *The Treatment of Pneumonoccic Pneumonia in the Adult* (Oakland: Permanente Foundation, 1948), 5.

3. Stevens, *In Sickness and in Wealth*, 177–178, 201–202; James H. Cassedy, *Medicine in America* (Johns Hopkins University Press, 1991), 125–129.

4. Cassidy, 125–129; Harold H. Bremers, M.D., "Diseases of the Skin," n.d.; Douglas Macomber, M.D., "The History of Plastic Surgery in Children's Hospital," 1979, Physician Typescripts, CHD Collection.

5. *Annual Report of the Colorado State Board of Health, 1940–1945* (Denver: State Office Building, 1946), 26–28.

6. Ibid., 32.

7. Ibid., 81.

8. Ibid.

9. Ibid., 37, 71–77.

10. Sydney A. Halpern, *American Pediatrics: The Social Dynamics of Professionalism, 1880–1980* (Berkeley: University of California Press, 1988), 111–112.

11. John C. Connell, M.D., Untitled medical history from 1942–1948, 1979, Physician Typescript, CHD Collection.

12. Ed Orsini, M.D., "History, Department of Pathology," March 1991, Physician Typescript.

13. Ibid.

14. Al Miller, M.D., "The Sands of Time" (history of staff through the 1950s), n.d., Physician Typescript.

15. Jean McMahon, M.D., "Physical Therapy — Occupational Therapy, Audio and Speech — D&E," probably part of the 1979 history, Physician Typescript.

16. Connell, Medical history, 1942–1948.

17. C. Richard Hawes, M.D., Untitled cardiology segment, 1979, Physician Typescript.

18. Connell, Medical history, 1942–1948.

19. Ibid.

20. *Forty-second Annual Report* (1952); *Forty-third Annual Report* (1953); *Annual Report* (1955–1956).

21. Quotes from Stevens, *In Sickness and in Wealth,* 175.

22. Connell, Medical history, 1942–1948.

23. Miller, "The Sands of Time."

24. Blaise Favara, M.D., "The Department of Pathology: Historical Notes," 1979, Physician Typescript; Connell, Medical history, 1942–1948.

25. David Akers, M.D., "Preface" (to a surgical history), 1979, Physician Typescript, CHD Collection.

26. Connell, Medical history, 1942–1948.

27. William R. Lipscomb, M.D., "A Real Dream," 1979, Physician Typescript, 1–4.

28. *Forty-sixth Annual Report* (1956), 12, 15.

29. *Red Apron* 1 (May 2, 1952): 1. This was a mimeographed newsletter published irregularly by the Auxiliary.

30. Mrs. Pearl Horner to Miss Bird, December 27, 1962; Richard Gottardi to Miss Hegvold, March 17, 1957; and Mr. and Mrs. Helmer Hendrickson to Children's Hospital Association, May 5, 1957; all in CHD Collection.

31. *Red Apron* 14 (July 1956): 2; and 1 (March 1952): 2–3.

32. Frances Wayne, "Bright Refuge," *Sunday Denver Post Empire Magazine* (October 6, 1949): 3.

33. Bill Slater, "Gus," *Point of View* (Spring 1980): 1–3. This was an in-house, irregular publication of the hospital.

34. "Physician Memories," December 1984, Physician Typescript, CHD Collection.

35. Connell, Medical history, 1942–1948.

36. Akers, "Preface," 8–9.

37. Miller, "The Sands of Time."

38. "Physician Memories."

39. Ibid.

40. Stevens, *In Sickness and in Wealth,* 177–178.

41. "Physician Memories."

42. Ibid.

43. Frances A. McDonough, "Class of 1952 Scrapbook," n.d., mimeograph in CHD Collection.

44. *Forty-third Annual Report*, 19; *Forty-fourth Annual Report* (1954), 4–5; Jolene Freimuth to Winifred Moss, "Summary Focus on the Division of Nursing," November 21, 1991, typescript in CHD Collection.

45. *Forty-fifth Annual Report* (1955), 21.

46. *Thirtieth Annual Report*, 63; "Charity Work, 1925–1942," Chart in *Thirty-fourth Annual Report* (1944), 29.

47. *Thirty-ninth Annual Report* (1949), 14; *Forty-eighth Annual Report* (1958), 13; *Forty-sixth Annual Report*, 12; Miss Pitt to Mr. Losh, interoffice memo, September 16, 1964, CHD Collection.

48. Miller, "The Sands of Time."

49. R. M. Dearing, "Annual Report of the Admissions Officer, 1938–1946," CHD Collection.

50. *Forty-third Annual Report*, 5

51. "Children's Hospital Building Program: The Oca Cushman Wing," pamphlet (Denver, 1958) in CHD Collection.

Chapter 5

Emergence of a Modern Institution, 1959–1975

Space in the new Oca Cushman Wing quickly filled. The 1960s and early 1970s marked rapid expansion of new subspecialties in fields previously falling under the general heading of internal medicine: pediatric cardiology, neonatology, and adolescent medicine. Hospital administrators struggled to meet seemingly insatiable demands for new equipment and adequate space.

They also realized the growing urgency of containing costs and providing more convenient, localized services. If more young patients could have their needs served promptly in outpatient clinics and sent home, rather than occupying hospital beds for long periods of time, Children's Hospital could cut costs for patients and use its space more efficiently. In addition, hospital leaders clearly recognized the necessity of further developing outreach activities not just within metropolitan Denver but throughout the Rocky Mountain region. Thus outpatient treatment, cost containment, and regional outreach became important objectives in the 1960s and 1970s.

At the beginning of this period far-sighted planners also expressed concern over long-term funding. As recently as 1940 nearly two-thirds of hospital revenues came from donations, endowments, and miscellaneous sources; twenty years later these sources yielded only 22 percent of the hospital's funding. In appeals for more generous donations, hospital leaders noted that "cost per patient per day" had risen to $41.81 by 1961. And accounting procedures were primitive by today's standards. Longtime volunteer Lenore Stoddart recalled that as late as the 1950s, bookkeeper Freida Kelly still used "large ledger books in which she entered every item of income and expense in a beautiful script."[1] The next fifteen years marked a fundamental shift in sources of income. State and federal appropriations and grants became crucial in both short- and long-range financial planning. The 1960s and early 1970s saw great changes in the level of federal government support for human services, including medicine. President John F. Kennedy evinced a new sense of concern about poverty, and it was during his abbreviated term in office that social critic Michael Harrington's acclaimed book, *The Other America* (1962), generated an enormous amount of support for federal assistance. It was left to Lyndon B. Johnson to coordinate the emergence of a patchwork of political programs that created billions of dollars for new social welfare programs.

The mid-1960s was the heyday of Johnson's Great Society programs. Medicare and Medicaid were cornerstones of an emerging national program to enhance access to medical care. Congress also funded a veritable cornucopia of federal grants to aid research and foster new clinics. To compete for funds, astute hospital administrators needed to learn the rules of grantsmanship. A hint suggesting just how "new" Children's Hospital personnel were in playing the game was the fact that a $1,000 research grant for cancer research from the Ladies Auxiliary of the Veterans of Foreign Wars merited a two-column story in the *Denver Post* in 1962.[2] In 1967 Children's Hospital director Norman Losh reported that "the main emphasis" of his office that year had been seeking federal and foundation grants.[3] A corner was turned; there could be no retreat to a simpler world. From that point forward one of the director's most critical tasks was to be aware of and conform to the rules and regulations of federal, state, and other institutional bureaucracies, while preserving a compassionate, humane atmosphere for patients.

Medical progress, public spending on health care, and the rising number of families with insurance challenged hospital planners to stay abreast of escalating middle-class demands for their children's health care. By 1980 over 92 percent of national hospital expenditures went through insurance, including government, Blue Cross, and other major insurance carriers.[4] In size and numbers of patients served, the hospital had come a long way in its first fifty years. From the converted private dwelling that contained only thirty-five beds in 1910, Children's Hospital had grown to be one of the nation's largest institutions in its category, with 255 beds. In 1955 only 15 percent of the nation's hospitals had more than 200 beds. By 1961 over 500 doctors were on the hospital's staff, and 550 employees provided full services to patients.[5] While a handful of staff physicians were engaged in clinical research, the majority were involved in private practice and provided basic health delivery services. There was routine cooperation with other hospitals. Children's maintained its autonomy and mission through a difficult period of growing pains and talk of merger with the University of Colorado Medical Center (UCMC).

The average hospital visitor in the early 1960s had little if any comprehension of these long-range concerns. He entered a beehive of activity. In 1963, during an average twenty-four-hour period, the hospital served 172 patients on a continuing basis and admitted thirty-seven new ones. There were 198 outpatient visits and thirty-seven physical therapy patients. Staff doctors conducted 800 laboratory examinations, performed thirty-one operations, and fifteen emergency room treatments. Other personnel served 901 meals, filled 572 pharmacy orders, and washed 3,705 pounds of laundry. Administrators were concerned that daily operating costs had jumped almost a third, from $6,798 to $9,958 between 1960 and 1963. Although more patients were being served, daily per-patient expenses had risen to $58.14. Thirty years later these costs appear almost ludicrously small. Even though he sensed a disturbing new trend, Director Losh's reaction to rising costs remained bullish, as he declared: "Instead of decrying costs, we at Children's would rather stress what that expenditure of monies has accomplished in terms of the increased efficiency of our medical staff, the surer treatment of patients, and the modernization of our hospital facilities. There is no substitute for progress. . . . And we must continue to bear its costs."[6] Later generations of doctors and hospital administrators would have to pull sharply back from this rhetoric of limitless expansion. By the mid-1960s one strategy for cutting costs was to shorten the average length of hospital stays and provide as many outpatient services as possible. Patients with long-term ailments primarily requiring rest and only occasional medical treatment were usually sent home. Administrators carefully monitored average lengths of stay per patient, and they directed inquiries when that figure increased.

The traditional model for an outpatient department until the second quarter of the twentieth century was one of episodic and acute care for the pediatric population, crowded clinics, outmoded facilities, and often indifferent personnel. These services were usually aimed at the children of low-income or indigent families.[7]

This situation was to change. Not only was medical/surgical care provided on an ambulatory basis highly cost-effective, it was now to be delivered with an aggressive dedication to the needs of the whole child: psychological, social, physical — and such care was not defined by socio-

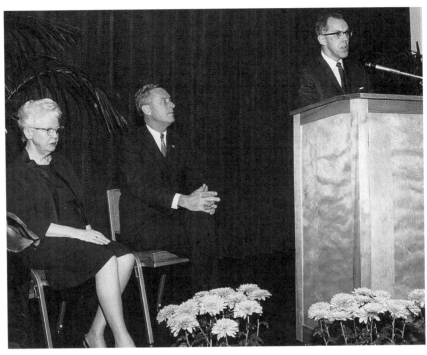

Mrs. Clara Van Schaack, past president of the board of directors, Governor John Love, and Norman Losh, executive director, at the Outpatient Building dedication.

economic status. New construction at Children's Hospital was designed for the efficient delivery of modern ambulatory services.

In 1967 Children's Hospital reached another milestone with the opening of a new $1.5 million outpatient building, mostly paid for by Hill-Burton Act federal funds. It was a five-story building that provided expansion for many specialty clinics: Development and Evaluation (D and E), Audiology and Speech Pathology, and others.[8] This epochal piece of federal legislation had numerous provisions, the most important of which was providing federal assistance for construction of new hospitals and clinics. Leaders at Children's Hospital applied for and received federal funding.

In September 1966 the Denver Department of Health and Hospitals received $1.5 million under a new Title V provision of the Social Security Act. These funds were to be used to provide basic health services for youngsters fourteen and under who otherwise would not receive them for reasons beyond their control. Several neighborhood health centers were established, and Children's Hospital received about $150,000 per year as its share. The experiment in this new means of delivering services to poor patients was named "Project Child."

Although Children's Hospital had given away millions of dollars' worth of health services to indigent patients over the years, it had never mounted a full-service health care program for low-income families. Since the 1920s the hospital had offered conventional outpatient services to neighborhood residents but had focused on nutrition and uncomplicated disorders. Patients took their turn on a first-come, first-served basis. Additional services to the community had also included a "well baby" clinic that offered instructions in caring for infants; it met three times a week. Hospital administrators could not justify providing more extended care because such a program could never come close to being self-supporting.

In the mid-1960s Children's Hospital administrators eagerly accepted the responsibility and challenges of Project Child. The funds were used primarily for staff salaries and some equipment. Project Child lasted about five years, until funds were terminated under the Nixon administration. At its peak in the early 1970s three pediatricians supervised its programs. They included Drs. Seymour Wheelock, director of community pediatrics, Hendrika Cantwell, Florence Uyeda, and Jean Haley, P.N.P., plus a dozen or so support personnel. In 1970, 3,500 children were enrolled in the program, and there were 10,000 visits to the new Ambulatory Pediatric Clinic in the Oca Cushman Wing. Although federal funding predictably was discontinued, Project Child initiatives evolved into much of the extensive Ambulatory Pediatrics Program currently in place at Children's Hospital. Patients of varied personal and financial backgrounds are cared for by means of the entire range of complex professional skills and technology implicit in the modern era of community and family-oriented pediatric medicine and surgery.

The mid-1960s also marked development of more services for adolescents and youths in their later teens. A grant from the Colorado Department of Institutions in 1963 permitted expansion of the new Child Guidance Center and the establishment of preventive medicine and psychiatric and psychological services to include emotionally disturbed youngsters. Dr. Wheelock guided many of the initiatives to assist healthy and troubled adolescents. This effort was consonant with the new frontiers of holistic care developed nationwide. The first generation of children brought up under the influence of Dr. Benjamin Spock was accustomed to freedom of expression and attention to emotional and psychological needs. The Youth Center in the remodeled isolation building, serving young people twelve to twenty-one year old, expanded its facilities in the form of a rooftop recreation center and a study room. Other clinics were established and rapidly expanded: the Well Baby Clinic and the Neurology, Ophthalmology, and Cardiac Clinics.

All of these initiatives required unprecedented infusion of funds. While the Auxiliary and other supporting groups continued fund-raisers, the proceeds constituted steadily decreasing percentages of operating expenses. The Auxiliary's fashion show at the Brown Palace netted more than $30,000 in 1967; but with annual operating expenses running nearly $4.5 million, this sum contributed to less than 1 percent of the total.[9] Inevitably Children's Hospital needed public funds, and it had to increase charges to patients. In 1960 Director Losh reluctantly announced a $1 per day increase in room rates. Ward patients would pay $19 per day, those in semiprivate rooms up to $21; a private room would cost up to $25. Early in 1961 Losh embarked on a personal crusade to eliminate waste. In late March he proudly informed the directors that by substituting plastic, reusable cups for paper cups in patients' rooms, the hospital had saved $316 over the previous five months. A week later Losh reported that purchasing agent Norman Wilmot had discovered a cheaper but adequate brand of paper towels. By converting to the less expensive brand, Losh anticipated $540 in annual savings.[10]

Considering ballooning hospital budgets in the 1990s, such cost savings might appear insignificant. Thirty years ago, however, the funds saved would buy far more goods and services. Even considering inflation, wage scales were quite low, particularly for semiskilled or unskilled personnel. Monthly salaries paid to supervisors for nursing service ranged from $440 to $480, and head nurses earned between $400 and $443. General-duty nurses received $320 to $350, licensed practical nurses $234 to $250. Orderlies earned only $173 per month, or about $1 per hour, and six housekeeping maids received a starting wage of $0.80 per hour.[11]

To preserve warmth and a people-oriented atmosphere at Children's, the efforts of volunteers were particularly critical. Even though their fund-raising efforts might provide smaller portions of capital outlay and operating budgets, their homemade toys, baked goods, musical performances, skits, holiday parties, and a wealth of other efforts brightened the days of young patients. Celebrities of all types, including sports figures, comedians, musicians, and other entertainers paraded through patients' wards and rooms on an almost daily basis. One volunteer recalled a visit by Bob Hope for one of the hospital's many dedication ceremonies in the 1960s. Hope learned that one patient was celebrating her sixteenth birthday. Sweeping into her room, he cried out, "Janet, sweet sixteen and never been kissed," then planted a big one on her!

In 1968 Children's Hospital organized one of the first amputee ski programs in the nation for children with limb deficiencies. Dubbed the Three Track Ski Club, it provided several dozen children enjoyable outings, first at Arapahoe Basin and later at Winter Park. Led by Drs. William Stanek and Duane Messner and Ms. Willie Williams, R.N., the youngsters invariably looked forward to these adventures in the snow. Volunteers helping the children never forgot the thrill of seeing young patients' faces glow when they achieved a run down the slopes. Snowy pratfalls usually caused more laughter than tears.

Program coordinators also paired children with Vietnam veterans recuperating from amputations at Fitzsimons Army Hospital. By all accounts the children and the veterans experienced the same beneficial psychological healing. Virginia McMurtry, who spearheaded fund-raising for the program, became an instructor herself. McMurtry recalled: "The children were in awe of the Vietnam heroes. And the veterans were in awe of the children. They thought that if a child could learn to ski, so can I. And, of course, the children wanted to be as courageous as the veterans. In the end, both learned self-sufficiency and experienced success. And the rest of us were rewarded from being with them. We caught the spirit."[12]

In 1970 the program moved to Winter Park. The ski program was so successful that it has become an integral part of the hospital's medical rehabilitation program, which introduces children with disabilities to leisure lifetime activities including golf, tennis, horseback riding, and river rafting. Participants range in age from eight to eighteen, and their disabilities include cerebral palsy, spina bifida, amputation, polio, muscular dystrophy, spinal cord injuries, a variety of orthopaedic conditions, and learning and motor disabilities.

The Evergreen Children's Hospital Guild organized an eight-week amputee golf program at the Hiwan Golf Club in 1969. Over the years the golf outings were also held at numerous other clubs in the region. In a

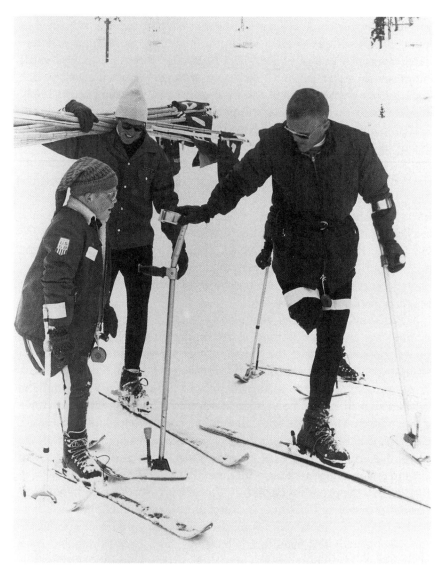

Young patient from Children's and a veteran from Fitzsimons Army Hospital enjoying participation in the Three Track Ski Club, one of the first amputee ski programs in the nation.

cooperative effort between the Children's Hospital Handicapped Sports Program and the Denver Public Schools' Boettcher School, bowling and archery were also available during the school year. Without question Children's Hospital became a leader in the nation in providing handicapped children access to normal activities. Hospital directors in other cities frequently requested information about Children's Hospital's initiatives in this area.

Patients and their parents expressed gratitude for care and services in many ways, mainly through letters of thanks and small gifts. Mr. and Mrs. Joseph L. Zangari of Denver had two daughters who received hospital care in the 1920s and 1930s. The family was unable to pay at the time, but in 1963 the parents sent in a $200 donation. Director Losh replied, "it is so gratifying to know that after all this time, you have remembered with appreciation." One couple was so moved by the valiant but unsuccessful efforts of Dr. C. Richard Hawes to save their daughter that they provided $300 as a memorial to her in 1962. Another couple recalled that when their seriously ill boy was admitted, "the first concern by the hospital was for Robert's illness. We were heartbroken to think that we might lose him. At no time during his long siege were we ever asked whether we could guarantee payment in any length of time. The personal warmth and concern for our worries has made the Children's Hospital an outstanding Hospital in Denver."[13] This couple repaid the Tammen Fund and added a contribution.

One of the buzzwords of the 1960s was "outreach," or serving the community. Children's began a series of public presentations, "The Family Forum," in which medical staff members discussed child health and parenting issues. Other initiatives developed that vastly improved the atmospheres in children's hospitals. One was a conscious effort to involve parents more directly in patient care. This mid-century development marked a rather dramatic attitudinal shift. According to one historian, as late as World War II "The hospitalized child . . . was considered essentially to be a biological unit, far better off without his parents who, on weekly or bi-weekly visiting hours, were fundamentally toxic in their effect, causing noise, generally disorderly conduct, and rejection by hospital personnel."[14] By the late 1950s visiting hours were becoming far more liberal, and numerous hospitals even allowed parents to "room in," or spend nights in their children's rooms. Medical leaders learned that parents were a vital positive influence on patient recovery. According to two other historians,

Charlene Holton, M.D.

Dr. Charlene Holton personified a new generation of doctors who combined pediatric research and caregiving opportunities at Children's Hospital in the late 1960s. Born in 1938, she graduated from the University of Miami Medical School in 1963. Dr. Holton accepted a residency in pediatrics at John Gaston Hospital in Memphis, followed by a two-month tour at the world-famous St. Jude's Hospital in the same city. At St. Jude's she had her first prolonged contact with children dying of leukemia and cancer. Her first feelings were acute depression over the daunting tasks confronting doctors, but soon she became encouraged by their progress in treating youngsters with radiation, surgery, and chemotherapy. She was awarded a research fellowship in oncology in 1966, and she subsequently decided to specialize in cancer care and research.

After a short stay as an assistant professor of pediatrics at the University of Tennessee, she came to Children's in 1968 to help organize the Oncology Clinic in cooperation with University Hospital. The clinic was soon treating 200 patients each month. Patients ranged from children with potentially curable diseases to those with only weeks or days to live. Many people asked Dr. Holton how she could continue to work creatively with dying children. She replied, "Most of what we do is manage the living child." In an interview she observed, "We feel if we can postpone death long enough, some bright person will find the answer, so we can treat the disease specifically. . . . After all, diabetes was always fatal until someone found insulin." Dr. Holton and several bright young colleagues applied successfully for a $500,000 research grant from the National Cancer Institute in 1972. By the early 1970s the Oncology Clinic at Children's was hard at work on research designed to find a cure for oncologic disorders, or at least to uncover techniques for helping patients lead active, happy lives until a cure would eventually be discovered.[15]

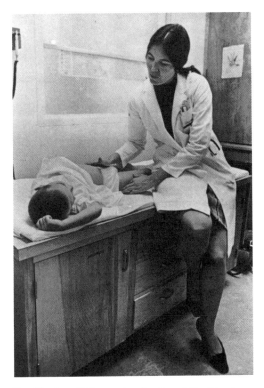

Dr. Charlene Holton, who developed the Oncology
Clinic in cooperation with University Hospital. Photo
by Bob Scott.

"Compared to hospital personnel, the parent typically enjoyed a unique
role by virtue of the child's trust and confidence in him. The parent can
serve not only to reassure, support and encourage his child, but also to
clarify and explain frightening procedures and occurrences. He brings a
familiar and immediate reality to some of the distressing fantasies of
hospital routine generated partly by the child's ignorance."[16]

Children's Hospital had in fact offered longer visiting hours to parents long before World War II, and hospital personnel enthusiastically
endorsed this new philosophy in almost every area at all hours. In addition,
parents were encouraged to share information and advice with hospital
personnel.

Another 1960s initiative that greatly enhanced the hospital's reputation for providing specialized services to the entire Rocky Mountain region

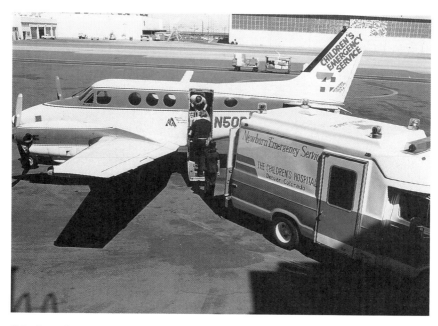

"Newborn Country U.S.A." became the slogan of the 1960s, and with the increased referrals to the Newborn Center, emergency transport services were developed to meet those needs.

was the Newborn Center, which opened under the direction of Dr. L. Joseph Butterfield on February 1, 1965. The center became known for innovative programs rather than for the latest in medical technology. For example, Butterfield was an advocate of a regional program for the delivery of perinatal care, Dr. Beverly Koops initiated a family care program, and Dr. Peter Honeyfield was assigned the Newborn Transport Program. Other examples were a regional perinatal education program and an expanded role in nursing called a neonatal nurse clinician. The center was one of the early advocates for affiliation with the University of Colorado Medical Center (UCMC) Department of Pediatrics, beginning in 1971 when Dr. Frederick Battaglia began making rounds at the Newborn Center.[17] When the Newborn Center began the practice of "shunting" excess neonatal referrals to UCMC, the alliance between the University and The Children's

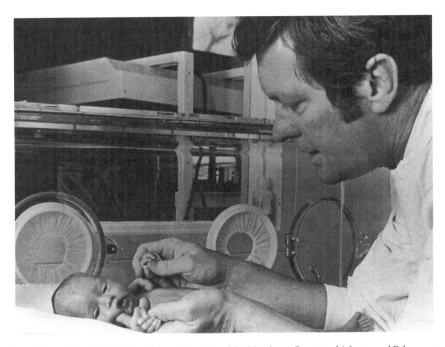

Dr. L. Joseph Butterfield, founder and director of the Newborn Center, which opened February 1, 1965.

Hospital was strengthened when Drs. Beverly Koops, Jim Lemons, and M. Douglas Jones, Jr., were recruited from the University to the Newborn Center staff at Children's.

In the late 1960s and early 1970s the Newborn Center developed a long reach, bringing in critically ill infants from Nebraska, Wyoming, New Mexico, and other states.[18]

In generating visibility and favorable publicity for Children's Hospital, the Newborn Center was a most valuable asset. In fact, the center and other highly specialized services did not significantly affect the geographic profile of patients served. By 1968 only 7.8 percent of all hospital patients served were from out of state, up from 5.3 percent a decade earlier. In 1968 more than four-fifths of all patients were from the Denver metropolitan area. Nevertheless, the Newborn Center was considerably more than a

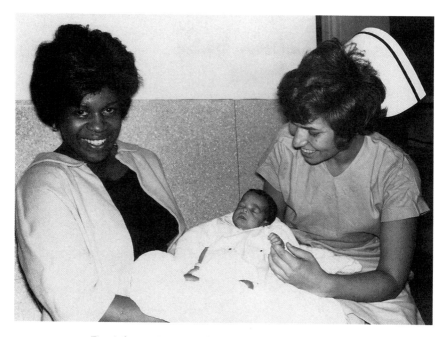

First infant patient going home from the Newborn Center.

short-term experiment or a publicity-generating device. Dr. Butterfield recalled its early years at some length:

> Since I was the only neonatologist, I recruited six pediatricians to take call every other month. In 1965 the technology of "intensive care" was limited. Mostly we cared intensely and worked a lot. . . . I was convinced that reaching out to the region we served was important, so I made plans to visit physicians and hospitals every month while I was off call. It was easy to pick the sites for visits; I called the doctors who referred patients to the Newborn Center and they were always willing to see me, if only for a cup of coffee. Others wanted me to discuss their patients at the hospital and frequently I was asked to give talks to the nurses and medical staff.
>
> Another reason for outreach was to remove myself from the Newborn Center, since I found myself coming to the hospital every day when I was in town. The mental and physical fatigue was enormous, so that I looked forward to getting away and seeing the people and the places in Newborn Country USA — a name that I conjured up during an interview with a writer for the Colorado Springs *Gazette*.[19]

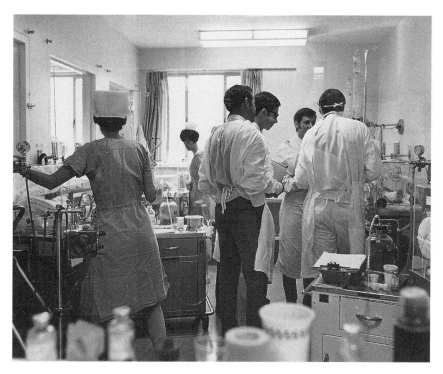

The success of the Newborn Center in 1965 led to crowded conditions and eventually the need to build a new center in 1975. Photo by Tom Masamori.

In 1966 Dr. Butterfield was a co-sponsor of a Ross Laboratories international conference on intrauterine transfusions. The following year the Aspen Conference for the Newborn was launched at the Aspen Institute for Humanistic Studies. That conference has continued to the present day and continues to attract practitioners from around the world; it is the oldest ongoing conference devoted to the newborn in the world. By 1975 the center admitted nearly 1,000 newborns a year.[20]

Yet another key outreach program was connected to the Newborn Center. At Children's the Perinatal Outreach Education Program (POEP) was first envisioned by Dr. Butterfield when the Newborn Center opened in 1965. The importance of this program quickly became apparent, as it became a means whereby referral hospitals could learn to enhance their stabilization care of critically ill newborns prior to transport, and Children's

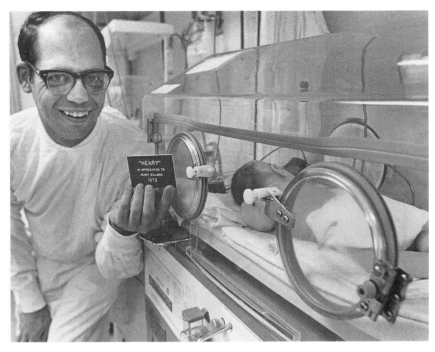

Henry Bollman, employee of Central Service, pictured here with an incubator he purchased and donated to the Newborn Center.

could gain access to referring hospitals to improve perinatal care in the Rocky Mountain/Western Great Plains region.

The POEP collaborated with Colorado General Hospital (CGH, now University Hospital) in the 1970s and St. Luke's from 1980 to 1989 to provide a full range of obstetrical and neonatal outreach services. Funding support was originally supplied in the form of seed money from the American Lung Association and the March of Dimes Birth Defects Foundation from 1973 to 1978. Further funding was provided by the Colorado Department of Health until 1982. Since 1982 Children's has provided program personnel salaries. Ongoing grant support has been obtained from a variety of private foundations, such as the McArthur Family Foundation, the Williams Family Foundation, the Little John Fund, and an anonymous donor in memory of Paulina Huff Carey.[21]

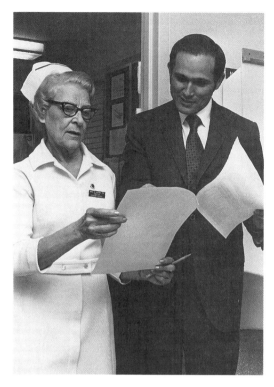

Francisco D. Sabichi, appointed executive director in 1969, with Sylvia G. Hoover, R.N., director of nursing, discussing ways in which administration and nursing could work together to provide quality patient care to the young patients and their families.

Dr. Jacinto Hernandez, a native of Peru, who trained in neonatal and perinatal medicine at the Children's National Medical Center in Washington, D.C., succeeded Dr. Butterfield as chairman of the Department of Perinatology in 1980. Dr. Hernandez's expertise as a clinician and bedside teacher won him the Gary Way Award for Outstanding Teaching from the teaching program at UCMC.

By the late 1960s, as Children's Hospital approached its sixtieth year of operation, administrators realized that another crucial decision-making period was at hand. It became evident that administrative and economic problems were mounting, but solutions were elusive. In 1970 recently appointed executive director Francisco D. Sabichi addressed "speculation that the nationally-famed institution had seen its better days." He noted that Children's was still trying to provide full services for young patients despite the nationwide trend toward specialization within pediatrics as in general medicine. Citing rumors of an imminent merger with UCMC Sabichi "was surprised to discover . . . [that] a number of people think we are about to close down."[22]

Children's Hospital remained the only hospital of its kind in the Rocky Mountain region, but other medical facilities were becoming increasingly competitive. Still, by the end of the turbulent 1960s Children's Hospital was outstanding in its innovative, up-to-date specialized services. Some twenty-six separate departments served inpatients; another sixteen provided outpatient treatment. Other departments and clinics besides the Newborn Center had bright futures, including the Oncology Department. These appeared well positioned to stay on the cutting edge of new medical breakthroughs.

Some of the problems facing Children's by the late 1960s affected other pediatric hospitals around the country. Increasing tensions arose within the pediatric profession between generalists and subspecialists. Since 1959 many subspecialties had emerged: preventive pediatrics, developmental pediatrics; adolescent medicine and gynecology; developmental pharmacology; and the epidemiology of congenital malformations, among others. Subspecialists' laboratories had yielded some impressive new medical advances. Analysis of sweat from children with cystic fibrosis, for example, facilitated earlier detection of this dangerous genetic disorder. New antimetabolites offered palliation of childhood cancers. Somatic cell cultures allowed prenatal diagnoses of dozens of genetic diseases. These advances were funded by a multiplicity of federal agencies, including the National Institutes of Health (NIH) and the National Science Foundation (NSF), which poured tens of millions of dollars into research. Public agencies were joined by dozens of private foundations supporting medical research.[23]

Amidst the excitement of emerging subspecialties and sponsored research, however, some practicing pediatricians and generalists felt devalued, even ignored. A number of pediatric generalists nationwide promoted more ambulatory services for children and adolescents. They focused considerable attention on psychosocial issues and a wide spectrum of newly identified behavioral disorders. They founded the Ambulatory Pediatric Association (APA) in 1960 and the Society for Adolescent Medicine

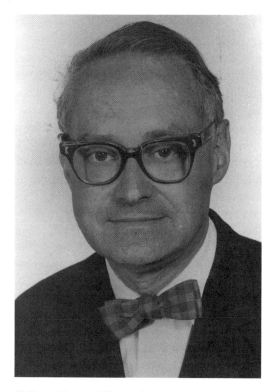

C. Henry Kempe, M.D., professor and chairman of the
Department of Pediatrics at the University of Colorado
School of Medicine from 1956 to 1973.

(SAM) in 1968. By the end of the decade many medical schools had
full-fledged departments offering training in adolescent medicine, behavioral pediatrics, and other psychosocial areas.[24] It was inevitable that many
ambitious pediatricians interested in generalized applications would have
mixed feelings. When Dr. Abraham Bergman, a founding member of the
APA, entered pediatrics in the late 1950s, he recalled rising tensions between generalists and subspecialists:

> The diagnostic and therapeutic tools used by the cardiologists, hematologists,
> endocrinologists and others have profoundly improved the care of children.
> Where the unique talent of all pediatricians used to be applied to the care of
> the newborn, now few of us "generalists" dare enter the sanctum of flashing
> lights, clicking machines, and hissing vapors.[25]

Other pediatricians who became generalists and entered family practice complained of the overly specialized directions of medical school training. Students spent far too much time studying cases, the insights from which they would rarely, if ever, apply. One generalist recalled that a young doctor from a prestigious training center complained to his former professor that while "he had been trained to race at Hialeah race track, he was now out pulling the chuck wagon like any other old dray horse."[26]

Tensions were evident between practicing generalists and research-oriented subspecialists at Children's Hospital of Denver. Some generalists complained that researchers reaped excessive economic rewards in terms of salary increases and that they received all the glory. These same doctors perceived a gradual dwindling of their status within the hospital's hierarchy. In contrast, some subspecialists believed that the generalists were resisting progress.

By the late 1960s acute financial problems were evident as well. The directors hired a management consulting team, Cresap, McCormick and Paget of New York, to investigate problems and recommend action. Early in 1969 the firm presented an incredibly thorough three-volume study, assessing the hospital's condition from every angle. Ironically, one financial analysis indicated that improvements in preventive and ambulatory medicine were resulting in lowering of the inpatient census. Total inpatient days peaked in 1963, at 62,465, then declined nearly 13 percent by 1967. Average bed occupancy dropped from 171 to 151 over the same period. During the 1960s the hospital downsized from 255 to 188 beds. Treatments provided by some departments declined even more precipitously. Ear, Nose, and Throat experienced the greatest drop-off, nearly 41 percent; the Surgical Department was not far behind, with a 25.6 percent decline.[27]

Many causes for the decline were happy ones for patients, including changed medical thinking and practice. Much of the inpatient census attrition was caused by the fact that many pediatric surgical procedures, formerly routine and forming a large percentage of earlier volume, were now seldom performed. Tonsillectomy and adenoidectomy was but one example. In addition, medical and surgical advances allowed more children with specific illnesses and injuries to be treated as outpatients. This was good news for families and children, even though it necessitated reorganization of traditional services.

Regional demographics also affected Children's patient load. Between 1960 and 1970 the total pediatric and adolescent population in the metropolitan region grew 25.4 percent. Denver, however, grew just 6.1 percent while the suburban population mushroomed 46.4 percent.[28] With a rapidly growing population in the region, new suburban hospitals opened and others expanded to include pediatric services. In 1960 only seven area hospitals offered acute-care pediatric services. By 1967 eleven of fifteen area hospitals provided those services; nine of them had modernized their pediatric units since 1961. During the 1960s hospital expansion exceeded demand, at least for inpatient needs. In the Denver region, bed occupancy averaged 69.3 percent in 1961, but it was just 63.2 percent six years later. While lower occupancy rates bothered hospital administrators throughout the region, leaders at Children's had additional cause for concern. The majority of new pediatricians in the region established offices and clinics in suburban areas. In many cases they referred patients requiring more than routine office services to a nearby hospital offering pediatric care. Children's was the only regional hospital devoted exclusively to children, but by the late 1960s it provided only 40 percent of pediatric care in the metropolitan area.[29] Of course the decentralization of services benefited pediatric patients, who did not have to go so far from their homes.

Despite the positive aspect of this trend, at least one insider at Children's Hospital envisioned little hope for cooperation and/or shared services that would achieve an ideal of quality pediatric care. In a confidential memorandum to the board of directors concerning the hospital's future, the board's first male president, Lawrence R. Reno, stated, "It is evident that we will not receive any assistance or cooperation . . . from the other hospitals in the area." He noted that St. Anthony's was constructing a new branch with pediatric beds in the Westminster-Northglenn area. Reno made a disturbing charge that St. Anthony's officials "have announced publicly to groups of physicians that they will not cooperate with Children's, which means they would probably be glad to see us go down the drain because they could then fill their beds more easily." He also noted that the Midtown Hospital Association had failed in its effort to better coordinate the distribution of pediatric beds in Denver hospitals.[30]

Health care industry competitiveness was reflected in even more worrisome financial reports. Operating losses mounted steadily in the 1960s. Although Children's Hospital lost nearly $745,000 in operations in 1963, revenues from endowments and gifts actually created a net surplus of $60,600. By 1967, however, a discouraging trend had emerged, showing increasingly large net losses each year. By 1967 Children's operating loss was over $1.3 million, and its net loss was $269,000. Projected losses for 1968 were even more alarming: operating losses approaching $1.5 million and a net loss of $423,000.[31]

The consultants admitted that their report "did not describe the major strong points . . . observed," but instead detailed the problems faced by the hospital. They acknowledged growing challenges in health care in the nation and region. Not only were government regulations increasingly cumbersome, but in the Rocky Mountain region cooperation between government agencies and medical services suppliers was almost totally lacking. Consequently there was considerable duplication of services and massive bureaucratic confusion. The Colorado State Health Department had recently established the Office of Comprehensive Health Planning, and the governor had appointed a State Health Planning Council. Earlier hospital administrators had set up the Midtown Hospital Association.

Each of these groups produced flowery position statements advocating enlightened cooperation and simplification of health care delivery. Unfortunately they generated little more than stacks of paper. Government agencies had little authority, and private groups often attempted to maneuver their competitors into making key concessions. Few hospital administrators envisioned long-term answers to the region's health care delivery dilemmas in the late 1960s. They were too busy solving immediate, day-to-day problems.

The consulting firm of Cresap, McCormick and Paget was pragmatic. Most of their recommendations focused on myriad internal problems at Children's Hospital. They particularly criticized management, in essence suggesting that it operated a multimillion-dollar institution like a "mom and pop" convenience store. Management positions were poorly defined, and the consultants urged development of a far more sophisticated and flexible administrative structure. For example, they were appalled at the lack of coordination in record keeping. When patients received services from several clinics, it took days before all charges were received in billing; this led to slow collections and bad debts. There was no single admissions form. Some clinics simply recorded patients' appointments on loose pieces of paper, then routinely destroyed them after a few weeks! Thus patients' medical records were either nonexistent or seriously incomplete. The consultants also concluded that administrators needed to learn cost accounting; inventory control was virtually absent, and purchasing was uncoordinated.[32]

The consultants also criticized personnel administration. There were too many small departments and clinics, inefficient wards, and nursing stations, and too many salaried doctors had been hired. The consultants questioned whether many of them attracted enough patients to pay their salaries. In striving to provide maximum service, some departments provided "unnecessary" levels of nursing and paid too much overtime; potential savings in nurses' salaries was $87,000 and nearly that much in doctors' salaries as well. Lack of coordination between surgery units and admissions personnel led to operations being booked without space available. Children's was misguided in trying to be all things to all people. The consultants declared that "meaningful, integrated planning does not exist at Children's Hospital, and it is providing services which are losing money and which may not be in Children's Hospital Association's best interest to provide." The consultants were amazed to learn that administrators had not even kept close watch on their service contract with Blue Cross. The last major contract had been negotiated in 1959, a full decade earlier. In general the consultants sensed an unwillingness on the part of decision makers to confront unpleasant economic realities, which were driven by events at the national level. Hospital leaders ignored the need for realistic rate increases for services rendered and refused to close inefficient and unprofitable clinics.[33]

Dorothy Heitler, a board member in 1968, recalled consternation and astonishment when Cresap, McCormick and Paget recommended that the women directors add men to the board. Until 1968 no men had served except in an advisory role. She recalled that many of the female members were powerful women whose children had left the nest. Financially secure, they had lots of time to devote to the hospital, and they thoroughly relished the opportunity to run a major institution. Many of the women enjoyed the hands-on work of helping children more than the dry, dull stuff of balance sheets and financial reports. But Mrs. Heitler conceded that adding men to the board in December 1968 created a more businesslike atmosphere. Walter Rosenberry III, who joined the board a few years later, recalled that many housewives still served when he first arrived. By the late 1970s most female members were business and professional women, significant in their own right.[34] Nevertheless, Lawrence R. Reno became the first male president the year membership was opened to men.

In 1980 Lenore Stoddart, longtime volunteer and president of the board at the time, recalled some of the "characters" who served before reorganization.

> Many of the "old guard" were still on the board then. I particularly recall with deep affection the late Mrs. Van Holt Garrett, a beautiful, regal lady who, during the baseball World Series, would attend board meetings with a small portable radio literally plugged into her ear. She would call out the score whenever one of the teams made a run. . . . In the early 1960s, board members served on a grounds committee, which conferred with tree-trimmers, nurserymen and the hospital gardeners. There was a decorating committee, which spent long hours deciding on colors for the walls and window coverings, in an effort to make the hospital a cheerful place.[35]

Some of the problems in administration were exacerbated by the inefficient hospital layout. Having expanded piecemeal, the hospital resembled a rabbit warren, mixing old and new structures, with small clinics in makeshift, temporary quarters and services randomly located. For example, the Newborn Center and the medical and surgical intensive care units were in three separate locations. The consultants urged coordination and physical consolidation of these and other clinical and administrative functions. Inefficient layouts and managerial confusion reinforced each other.[36]

Beyond hospital walls the consultants urged greater cooperation with other health care providers in the region. But the most important single recommendation involved some form of merger with the University of Colorado Medical Center (UCMC). The report read: "Currently, both institutions are duplicating programs and services to strengthen their positions in the health care system and to meet internal program requirements; these developments have resulted in the continued fragmentation of services and increased health care costs to the community." The consultants urged Children's to adopt one of two alternative plans to merge with UCMC. The first, "less radical" proposal was that Children's would remain at its present location, "a free-standing pediatric hospital physically separate but academically affiliated with UCMC." The preferred, recommended "radical" alternative was to consolidate pediatric health care programs at one institution. Children's would build a new facility on the UCMC campus, "expanding patient care, education and research programs through an institutional and academic affiliation with the UCMC School of Medicine."[37]

Lenore Stoddart

Mrs. Stoddart personified the term "volunteer." Her first recollection of Children's Hospital was at age eight, when she had a tonsillectomy. At age sixteen she started as a volunteer, running errands for Mrs. Cushman. In the 1950s she assisted Children's accountant Freida Kelly, and performed many other tasks. She helped nurses undress injured children. At other times she might read stories to a child who had undergone eye surgery. After the Auxiliary was founded, she worked in the gift shop or snack bar. She often took the book cart from ward to ward, tempting young readers.

As her own executive skills developed, Stoddart was entrusted with the Tammen Visiting Physicians and Surgeons Fund, which provided token honorariums for doctors serving the hospital under certain circumstances. Elected to the board of directors in 1960, she was chosen president in 1968 and served during the crucial years when the board was reorganized and men were added.

The consultants reinforced ideas that had been under consideration by spokespersons from the two institutions for at least four decades. In the mid-1920s a handful of doctors believed that merger with the brand new UCMC (opened in 1924) would enhance the image of Children's Hospital and no doubt allow them to refocus their own careers by creating more professional opportunities. They ran into a buzz saw of opposition from the executors of the Tammen estate. According to both Mrs. Tammen and the trustees, the hospital's biggest benefactor had always wanted the hospital to focus exclusively on the care of children rather than research. A trustees' statement in 1927 made their position clear: "In compliance with a request for our views on the proposal to affiliate the Children's Hospital with the Medical Department of the University of Colorado, we are compelled to state that an affiliation of this nature is not, in our opinion, advisable."[38] An unstated, but clearly implied fear of the women directors in the 1920s was that Denver children would be subjected to some danger of "experimentation." These same fears were often expressed by female directors at children's hospitals elsewhere in the country.

Four decades later Cresap, McCormick and Paget's merger recommendation was to appear both intelligent and logical — to outsiders. In fact, leaders at the respective institutions, state lawmakers, the Denver Regional Council of Governments (DRCOG), the regents at the University of Colorado, and other key players became deeply involved in negotiations that continued into the 1990s. Realities were far more complex than they appeared on the surface. Large and powerful factions and interest groups at both institutions opposed a merger. Department chairmen and heads of independent clinics feared elimination or reduction in size of units and/or potential demotions. In addition, mergers of clinics and departments threatened professional fees of doctors at UCMC who provided services to private patients. Other problems surfaced as the two institutions continued a lengthy, troubled courtship.

By the middle of the 1970s the "romance" had taken many complex twists and turns, and plans had come tantalizingly close to fruition. During early merger talks, progress appeared steady. Late in 1970 a formal affiliation agreement was reached. Representatives of the two institutions created a Joint Coordinating Committee to exchange information, initiate planning, and make recommendations to the governing bodies of their respective organizations.[39]

Children's negotiators sensed, however, that to achieve affiliation they would have to make the most critical concessions and compromises. In November 1970 board chairman Lawrence R. Reno expressed frustration over submitting "at least the eleventh draft presented by the Children's Hospital Negotiating Committee to the UCMC." There was no debate over which institution would make the most capital commitments. Children's Hospital envisioned constructing a new, modern hospital across Colorado Boulevard from UCMC. The facility would cover several city blocks and would be physically connected to UCMC by a walkway over Colorado Boulevard, or a tunnel underneath it.

In May 1971 Children's Hospital hired professional fund-raisers to begin an intensive thirteen-month capital fund drive. A month later negotiators discussed engineering specifications regarding the connecting bridge or tunnel between the two institutions and other very specific plans. They also planned meetings with the Denver City Planning staff and other public officials. In June 1972 the board at Children's voted unanimously in favor of moving to the site across Colorado Boulevard from UCMC, "provided that land acquisition, plans and specifications for the new facility and financial matters regarding the resolution are satisfactory."[40] Financial planners estimated the capital outlay at between $15 million and $25 million, including land acquisition. By the end of 1972 representatives of Children's had acquired several parcels of real estate — no small achievement in a neighborhood containing a number of private homes.

Negotiations floundered on the practical issues involved with affiliation in the fall of 1972. By late September negotiators for Children's expressed open dismay over endless bureaucratic complications raised by UCMC officials. They sensed that UCMC negotiators were dragging their feet. Hospital administrator Francisco Sabichi complained to Dr. Robert Aldrich, vice president for health affairs at UCMC, that "in planning and commitment, the Children's Hospital is several steps ahead of the University of Colorado Medical Center." He urged firm commitments from UCMC "at the earliest possible date."[41] By late 1972 Children's Hospital had already sponsored several feasibility studies at a cumulative cost of $135,000. Inflation concerned the directors; each month's delay in starting construction of the new hospital added $100,000 to costs. Children's had planned to authorize detailed architectural plans early in October, but Sabichi had to rescind the invitation.[42]

As more and more study groups and mid-level administrators examined merger issues, complications multiplied. Close examination of the relationship among UCMC, Colorado General Hospital (CGH), and state and local officials revealed that institutional mandates and structural issues were extremely complex. As a state hospital CGH had a legal obligation to provide indigent care, and it also received state funds. State officials, therefore, were interested chiefly in providing competent medical care at the least possible expense. In the late 1960s and early 1970s increasing numbers of medical students attended UCMC, and used CGH for teaching and clinical experience. Hence, staff members at CGH were increasingly research oriented. State legislators worried that the public health care function of CGH was being neglected and that medical students and supervising physicians paid full attention only to the more "interesting" cases.

Children's Hospital board members voiced similar concerns. CGH was under intense external scrutiny, and when an unanticipated financial crisis emerged early in 1973, University of Colorado president Frederick P.

Thieme notified the CU regents that, because of negative legislative attitudes toward operations at CGH, UCMC had "been fighting for its life in
recent months." The university had requested a $3.4 million supplemental
appropriation to cover unanticipated costs but had received only $1.8
million, leaving a $1.6 million shortfall. Ironically, when merger discus-
sions began in the late 1960s, Children's Hospital had been in severe
financial straits, with CGH on solid financial footing. Now the positions
were reversed.[43]

Negotiators for Children's Hospital had demonstrated both patience
and remarkable restraint. Clearly there were basic differences in outlook
between professionals at the two institutions. If clinics and departments
merged, doctors had to work together, and in some cases it was like mixing
oil and water. One observer cited difficulties in merging the two radiology
departments. The unit at Children's provided sound, patient-oriented
service. In contrast at CGH the emphasis was more upon theory and
research. Since residents needed to obtain maximum education during
their rotations, few would choose to work under the radiologists at Children's. Turf battles might erupt far down the line, even within nurses'
quarters and offices of supporting staff.[44]

The outlook for merger appeared even gloomier in 1974. A report to
the CU regents in March indicated that CGH might experience an annual
deficit in excess of $3 million. In contrast — and thanks in part to the highly
successful fund-raising campaign for construction of the new hospital —
Children's had net earnings in 1973 of $780,000. Board members at Chil-
dren's worried that as a consequence of the merger their endowment funds
might simply be swallowed up in UCMC's bureaucratically administered
public appropriation. The regents feared that if CGH moved its 100 pediatric
beds, they would dig themselves into an even deeper hole. With high fixed
costs and shrinkage of beds from 450 to as few as 290, escalating per-patient
costs could plunge CGH into a crisis of economics and prestige.[45]

Nevertheless, leaders at Children's made another concerted effort to
put the merger over the top. In mid-summer 1974 Mrs. Norman Davis,
president of the board, pinpointed both the concerns and hopes of her
associates. She observed that a negative by-product of the stalled talks was
the drain on existing programs: "Many professional programs and plans
have been held in abeyance for many months. . . . The indecision has had
an enervating effect on the entire hospital family." Still she hoped that the
merger could occur if both sides rededicated themselves to the task: "We

don't wish to hear why this concept won't work, we expect our staff to make it work."[46]

Then the regents effected a seemingly dramatic turnaround and publicly committed to merger on July 18, 1974. There was, however, one major caveat: merger would depend on approval by the Colorado legislature and its "necessary financial support." In retrospect this "commitment" was an empty gesture. Less than a month later a state official informed university president Roland Rautenstrauss that reports of the merger caused concern at the capitol. Budget overruns at CGH would not be overlooked or forgiven so quickly, and he believed it would take three or four years to straighten out the mess.[47] Other bad news plagued negotiators' efforts. In early December 1974 the Boettcher Foundation announced withdrawal of a million-dollar commitment to the building fund, at least "until the program can be well defined."[48] There was also significant public opposition to the relocation plan. For several years representatives for Children's Hospital had been purchasing land in the proposed relocation area just west of UCMC. Their discussions with local officials had been reasonably well publicized, and they had suggested meetings with neighborhood groups as early as 1971. Nevertheless, early in 1975, local property owners united in opposition to the relocation of Children's. At a public meeting at the Denver Botanic Gardens on February 25, over 100 people opposed the move, protesting that it would "disrupt a very pleasant and very stable residential area." The controversy simmered until later in the spring. A mayoral election was scheduled for May, and several candidates lashed out at the hospital. Both the incumbent mayor, William H. McNichols, and his opponent, Dale Tooley, who later became a director of the hospital, opposed relocation. Vehement public opposition discouraged those pushing for relocation, and this new hurdle indirectly affected the merger itself. Negotiators for both sides postponed implementing the combined program agreement of December 1974.[49]

Board president Mrs. Davis attempted to put the best face on it, praising the sincere efforts of both sides' representatives and lauding progress in coordinating joint efforts in teaching and research. She allowed that, in 1975, "Maybe the time was not right," yet she held out hope for the future. The attitude of one official at UCMC was decidedly less benign. He charged that opposition of Congress Park neighbors was only an excuse by internal opponents of the merger to pull out: "Had there been sufficient

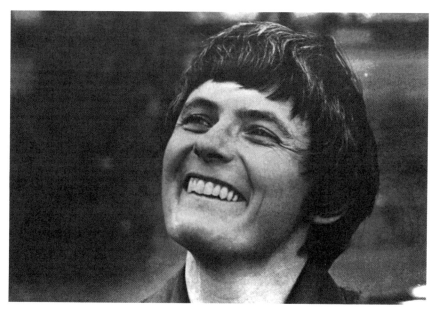

Dr. Ann Kosloske, one of the few women pediatric surgeons in the United States in the early 1970s.

impetus on behalf of both institutions, some other satisfactory physical location could have been found."[50]

As the merger issue dominated board meetings and high-level consultations among administrators, Children's continued providing service to tens of thousands of children each year. In the late 1960s and early 1970s, lay administrators worried about the downward spiral of inpatients. In 1966 the hospital served 11,956 inpatients; numbers declined steadily over the next eight years, and in 1974 only 7,539 inpatients were recorded. Happily, the average length of stay had declined as well to less than five days per patient. In the latter year just over 37,000 patient days were recorded, a decline of more than 25,000 since 1967. On the other hand, outpatient services boomed, with just under 84,000 visits in 1974. The reasons for declining inpatient numbers were obvious. Medical technology and new antibiotics were helping cure serious illnesses much more efficiently, and more illnesses could be handled less expensively on an outpatient basis. In addition, there was far more competition for inpatient

Dr. Ann Kosloske

Growing up in a conservative midwestern city in the 1950s, Dr. Ann Kosloske found little encouragement for young women who aspired to become doctors, so she kept her ambition largely under wraps. In fact, her family considered her notions "wild ideas" but she persisted nonetheless. She recalled that at Marquette University it was not "socially advantageous" for a woman to be in pre-med, so she never told dates what her major was.

At Marquette School of Medicine she found surgery fascinating, and her internship at Johns Hopkins gave her a final push. She did six years of residency and general surgery at the University of Cincinnati Hospital Group, where in her final year she served as chief resident and instructor. After a year's stint split between Europe and India, she returned to a two-year fellowship in pediatric surgery at Cincinnati Children's Hospital. Shortly after her return to the United States, a near epidemic of necrotizing enterocolitis influenced the direction of her research interests.

In 1973 Dr. Kosloske ended thirteen years of training and accepted a position at Children's Hospital in Denver. Quickly moving into the Department of Pediatric Surgery at Children's, she also joined the clinical faculty of the Department of Surgery at UCMC. In her view she enjoyed "the best of both worlds." Amazingly she still had time to pursue her hobbies of skiing, golf, general fitness, and classical piano. Without question her career provided a sterling example for other ambitious young women exploring professional opportunities in the early 1970s.[51]

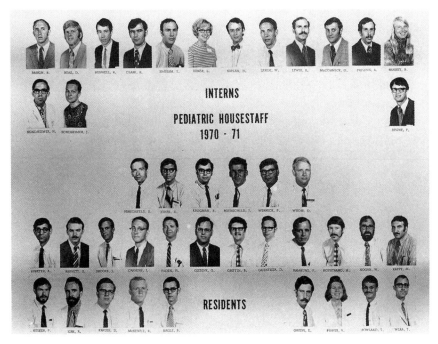

Children's provided clinical medical education to students from the University of Colorado Medical School. Pictured here are members of the pediatric house staff in 1970–1971. Many of these physicians remained in the Denver metropolitan area and have been influential in the pediatric medical community.

referrals in the metropolitan region, as other hospitals introduced or up-graded pediatric services.[52]

Thanks in part to the streamlining of the late 1960s and the increase in both private and public funding in the early 1970s, Children's Hospital operated on a balanced budget by the mid-1970s. Hospital leaders presided over an institution that had changed significantly over the previous fifteen years. Serving young patients remained the unquestioned top priority, but the hospital had wisely recruited a number of young physicians who were committed to pioneering research.

The 1974 annual report devoted lengthy sections to research and graduate education at Children's Hospital. It cited a $500,000 award to the Oncology Unit from the National Cancer Institute, along with significant research contributions by physicians in surgery, gastroenterology, the Newborn Center, and several other departments. There was progress in graduate education. Resident physicians were finally responding to a more lively intellectual climate; by 1974 twenty-four first-year residents and forty-two second- and third-year residents were rotating among CGH, UCMC, and Denver General Hospital (DGH).

On the other hand the collapse of merger talks with UCMC left hospital leaders in a vacuum. For almost a decade they had considered Children's future primarily within the context of merger. As one insider viewed the conundrum late in 1975, "There really was no plan B." As the twentieth century entered its last quarter, hospital leaders asked themselves, "What do we do now?" Merger with UCMC would indeed eventually occur, but no one in the late 1970s could peer that clearly into the future. In the meantime Children's Hospital struggled to redefine its mission while maintaining its autonomy and quality of care in a rapidly changing regional market and profession. These myriad challenges severely tested the resolve of the entire staff and all of the outside supporters who believed in Children's Hospital.

Notes

1. *Fifty-first Annual Report* (1961), 2, 5; Lenore Stoddart, "Prologue," January 22, 1980, manuscript in CHD Collection.

2. *Denver Post*, November 7, 1962.

3. *Fifty-seventh Annual Report* (1967).

4. Short-term private hospitals increased expenditures fourfold from 1950 to 1965, with a high at $9.1 billion nationwide. In 1940 only 9 percent of the U.S. population had health insurance; in 1975 numbers peaked at 82.5 percent. National spending on medical care continued to rise astronomically, to over 14 percent per capita annually after establishment of Medicare and Medicaid in 1965. See Rosemary Stevens, *In Sickness and in Wealth: American Hospitals in the Twentieth Century* (New York: Basic Books, Inc., 1989), 256–259; and Rickey L. Hendricks, *A Model for National Health Care: The History of Kaiser Permanente* (New Brunswick: Rutgers University Press, 1993), 206–207.

5. Stevens, *In Sickness and in Wealth*, 203, Table 9.2.

6. *Fifty-third Annual Report* (1963).

7. These trends were not unique to Denver. The much older Children's Hospital of Boston, affiliated with Harvard Medical School, also added an eleven-story building for outpatient care. As a further example of the shift from inpatient to outpatient care, hospital days at the Boston hospital decreased 45 percent and total admissions by 40 percent, while medical outpatient services increased 80 percent. See Clement A. Smith, M.D., *The Children's Hospital of Boston: "Built Better Than They Knew"* (Boston and Toronto: Little, Brown and Co., 1983), 247.

8. A resurgence of outpatient services and pressure to create regional multihospital systems also marked national efforts to meet escalating demands for service and runaway costs.

The Hill-Burton Hospital Construction Act of 1946 was a major federal thrust at voluntary regional planning at the state level. A second major federal effort to support the growing medical establishment, while keeping control at the state and local levels, was the rapid increase in funding for the National Institutes of Health (NIH), whose research budget rose from $180,000 in 1945 to $46.3 million only five years later. Stevens, *In Sickness and in Wealth*, 201; Paul Starr, *The Social Transformation of American Medicine* (New York: Basic Books, Inc., 1981), 342–343.

9. "Historical Overview: The Department of Psychiatry and Behavioral Sciences, The Children's Hospital," ca. 1991, mimeograph in CHD Collection; *57th Annual Report.*

10. Losh to Members of the Medical Staff, interoffice memorandum, October 10, 1960; Losh, "Weekly Report to the Board of Directors," March 30, 1961; and Ibid., April 7, 1961; all in CHD Collection.

11. "Hospital Personnel Data," ca. 1961, mimeograph in CHD Collection.

12. Photocopy of "Handicapped Sports Defies Disability," brochure in CHD Collection, 7.

13. Mr. and Mrs. Joseph Zangari to Children's Hospital, December 2, 1963; Losh to Mrs. Zangari, December 5, 1963; Mr. and Mrs. Chester Turpin to Dr. Hawes, December 18, 1962; all in CHD Collection.

14. Andrew D. Hunt, "On the Hospitalization of Children: An Historical Approach," *Pediatrics* 54 (November 1974): 542

15. *Denver Post Contemporary Magazine,* November 30, 1969, 6–8; Dr. James Todd, "Clinical Science With a Heart: The History of Research at The Children's Hospital, 1910–1990," 1991, typescript, CHD Collection, 7–8.

16. H. E. Rie and B. J. Grossman, "Parent Education in a Children's Hospital," *Clinical Pediatrics* 30 (February 1991): 102.

17. L. Joseph Butterfield, M.D., memorandum to Ms. Winifred Moss, August 3, 1993, CHD Collection.

18. *Fifty-ninth Annual Report* (1969), 8.

19. L. Joseph Butterfield MD, memo to Mark S. Foster, July 14, 1993, CHD Collection.

20. *Children's Hospital Association: A Program for Future Development* (New York: Cresap, McCormick and Paget, 1969), A-24; *Denver Post* advertising supplement, ca. 1976.

21. Susan Clarke, R.N., to Margaret Lister, July 19, 1993, CHD Collection.

22. *Rocky Mountain News,* February 15, 1970.

23. Thomas A. Cone, M.D., *History of American Pediatrics* (Boston: Little, Brown and Co., 1979), 229, 231.

24. Sydney A. Halpern, *American Pediatrics: The Social Dynamics of Professionalism, 1880–1980* (Berkeley and Los Angeles: University of California Press, 1988), 129.

25. Ibid., 136.

26. Ibid., 137.

27. *A Program for Future Development*, II-4; *Children's Hospital of Denver: Audit of Management and Operations* (New York: Cresap, McCormick and Paget, 1969), Exhibits II-A and II-B. These statistics were not unique. Children's Hospital of Boston showed even more dramatic declines. See Smith, *Children's Hospital of Boston*, 247.

28. *A Program for Future Growth and Development*, Exhibit A-1.

29. Ibid., A-6, A-23, III-6.

30. Lawrence R. Reno, "Confidential Memorandum" to Board of Directors, Children's Hospital, ca. November 1970, CHD Collection, 2.

31. *Audit of Management and Operations*, Exhibits II-A and II-B.

32. Ibid., III-5, IV-8.

33. Ibid., IV-3, IV-1, IV-7–8.

34. Mrs. Dorothy Heitler, interview by Winifred Moss, May 22, 1992; Walter S. Rosenberry III, interview by Moss, August 15, 1991.

35. Lenore Stoddart, "Prologue," January 22, 1980, manuscript in CHD Collection, 4.

36. *Audit of Management and Operations*, III-15, V-11, 12.

37. Ibid., IV-40, with cover letter to Mrs. John T. Stoddart, Jr., January 23, 1969.

38. Trustees Under the Last Will and Testament of H. H. Tammen, Deceased, to the Board of Directors, Children's Hospital Association, ca. 1927, CHD Collection.

39. "Programmatic and Economic Feasibility for Relocating Children's Hospital to the UCMC Campus," ca. 1973, mimeograph in CHD Collection, 1.

40. Francisco D. Sabichi to Dr. Robert Aldrich, March 6, 1972; Brennan to Robert W. Bechtel, June 30, 1972; mimeographed press release, July 6, 1972; all in CHD Collection.

41. Sabichi to Aldrich, September 26, 1972.

42. Aldrich to Sabichi, October 13, 1972; "Meeting Between Board of Regents of the University of Colorado and the Executive Committee of the Children's Hospital," February 28, 1973, mimeographed notes, 4.

43. Ibid.

44. "Radiology and Pathology," ca. October 1974, mimeograph in CHD Collection.

45. Francisco D. Sabichi to unknown, March 25, 1974, photocopy; Minutes, Meeting of Children's Hospital Directors and Board of Regents, University of Colorado, April 17, 1974; Mrs. Charles G. Gates to Lawrence Reno, June 10, 1973; all in CHD Collection.

46. Mrs. Norman B. Davis to Dr. Dale Atkins, July 16, 1974, CHD Collection.

47. Francisco D. Sabichi to staff member, July 18, 1974; Petrone to Rautenstrauss, August 12, 1974; both in CHD Collection.

48. John C. Mitchell to Mrs. Leslie F. Davis, December 5, 1974, CHD Collection.

49. Thomas M. Rauch to Mrs. Norman Davis, April 23, 1975; Tooley to Mrs. Norman Davis, May 15, 1975; both in CHD Collection.

50. "Minutes, Joint Meeting — Board of Directors — Board of Regents, August 14, 1975; Conrad M. Riley, M.D., to Mrs. Norman Davis, August 16, 1975, CHD Collection.

51. *Point of View* (August 1974): 3–5.

52. "Information given to L. Reno, May 2, 1975," mimeograph; *Annual Report* (1974), 15; "The Children's Hospital Association, Contributions and Investment Income, 1966–1974," ca. 1975, mimeograph; all in CHD Collection.

Chapter 6

Promises and Perils of Modernization

As Children's Hospital entered the last quarter of the twentieth century, many unsettled questions remained. Some issues seemed beyond the control of hospital administrators yet continued to consume much of their time and effort. Spiraling health care costs, the growing complexities of dealing with private insurers and government agencies, increasing numbers of indigent families, more competition in attracting paying patients — these and other problems challenged hospital leaders. They resolved some issues at the regional and local levels. In 1975 the issue of merger with the University of Colorado Medical Center was temporarily abandoned; however, by 1991 an affiliation was finally achieved. Although the two institutions remained detached physically, by 1991 a number of services and departments were combined.

Having committed to independence in the mid-1970s, Children's Hospital embarked on a major building program. Although competition with other hospitals intensified in the late 1970s and 1980s, Children's more than held its own. Between 1975 and 1990 inpatient numbers began to grow again, and outpatient visits nearly doubled. Facilities once again became crowded, and hospital leaders faced a renewed challenge in providing sufficient space. Despite these pressures hospital leaders remained focused on their central objective: giving care to children. Striving to create an attractive, nurturing working environment, they encouraged professional growth and development. They boasted a team of nearly 2,000 employees in 1990. Through turmoil, crisis, and growth, the focus was always on the child.

Few involved in merger negotiations in the mid-1970s expected a quick, formal affiliation of Children's Hospital with the Pediatrics Department at UCMC. Having issued optimistic and premature statements about progress in the past, spokespersons for both sides now were cautious and anxious to avoid public relations gaffes. In fact, negotiators conveyed considerable pessimism. In 1976 the dean of UCMC's School of Medicine publicly admitted to Children's Hospital executive director Francisco D.

Norman Wilmot

Few employees served Children's Hospital longer than did Norman Wilmot. In 1930 jobs were scarce, particularly for young men with little experience, but the enterprising young man applied for a two-week "temporary" opening for an orderly and was hired. In his own words, "I was such a sweet young kid that they kept me on." Quite an understatement — he retired in January 1978 after forty-seven years of service, two years more than the legendary reign of Oca Cushman.

Wilmot's trademark was versatility; he performed many tasks and shifted duties as the hospital changed. One of his important early duties was chauffeuring Mrs. Cushman about in her two-door coupe. He performed duties as basic as folding diapers and also worked as an orderly in surgery, a painter, carpenter, and at other jobs: "I've done just about everything here but run the place," he proclaimed in an interview. In the 1950s he took on the duty of buying supplies needed by the hospital, "making sure that everything necessary for running the hospital, from pencils to surgical instruments, was where it was needed." The job became increasingly important and complex. He became purchasing agent, and later his title was changed to director of purchasing.

With an office tucked away at the back of the first floor, Wilmot managed to achieve close ties to workers all around the hospital. Always ready to lend a hand in any emergency, he recalled the camaraderie uniting employees and volunteers: "We were really a family."[1]

Sabichi that conflict between departments revolved around familiar issues: UCMC personnel focused on the alleged disinterest in research on the part of many practitioners at Children's Hospital. For their part some department heads at Children's worried that "academic types" at UCMC would ignore or dehumanize patients. A few administrators at UCMC overtly resisted further efforts at cooperation. In May 1976 Dr. Thomas E. Starzl,

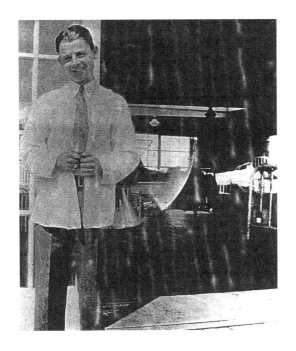

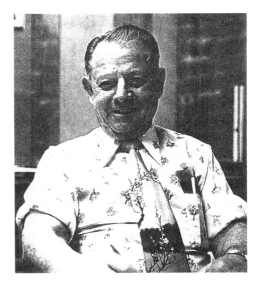

Norman Wilmot pictured here as a young man and at the time of his retirement in 1978 after forty-seven years of service.

chairman of surgery at UCMC, imperiously announced plans to terminate affiliation of his unit with its counterpart at Children's in a year's time.[2]

Negotiators sensed an impasse, and they agreed to bring in outside experts to help untangle the knots. Unbiased reviewers perceived the same conflicts. A consultant from the Mayo Clinic early in 1977 observed personality clashes between "certain members" of the surgery units: "These differences unfortunately became public, resulting in a disruption in the training experience of the residents . . . and eroding or injuring the reputation of the hospital." A review committee of several surgeons from the University of Pittsburgh Medical School cited long-term misunderstandings as the root cause of frayed relations between the two institutions. Furthermore Children's was the loser. The committee reported, "There is no question that events of the last six or seven years have been disruptive and detrimental to the reputation of Children's Hospital."[3]

Nevertheless the University of Pittsburgh consultants insisted that Children's and UCMC had much to contribute to the long-range success and growth of the other. Certain units at Children's Hospital, such as the Burn Unit, could stand on their own. In addition, some services at Children's Hospital were already effectively integrated with UCMC: "The perinatal program . . . is outstanding and a monument to full integration with the university and other resources in the community." Equally important, although a few individuals in both institutions feared invasions of their turf, the consultants found through interviews dozens of people on both sides who welcomed cooperation. In the late 1970s, however, negotiations concerning possible "reaffiliation" of the surgical departments were a microcosm of the problems inherent in combining two proud institutions. Dr. Jack H.J. Chang, chairman of general pediatric surgery at Children's, worried about domination by UCMC. He stated in July 1978, "I fear that Drs. Starzl and Lilly do not understand the difference between a cooperative venture and assumption of total control." Dr. Robert W. Hendee, a "neutral observer" representing Denver Neurological Associates, confirmed Chang's view: "It sounds more as if there is to be a takeover rather than a renegotiated reaffiliation." Hendee believed that Children's Hospital should stand firm in protecting its concerns.[4]

Despite misunderstandings and personal conflicts among some department heads, progress was made. In early 1979 Dr. Richard W. Olmsted, medical director at Children's Hospital, observed that positive gains had been achieved in critical care, continuing education, the ambulatory program, neurology, pulmonology, and perinatology. A joint committee on critical care resolved that "disposition of original patients needing intensive care [should] depend on practical consideration of institutional expertise rather than allocation or protocol."[5]

The 1980s saw cooperation in many areas between the two institutions, but some old problems remained. Basic philosophical differences that thwarted merger in the early 1970s were not yet resolved. By the late 1980s Denver-area health care officials realized that doctors at each hospital were "miles apart philosophically" and were unwilling to move much closer together. Nevertheless, in November 1988 top officials from both institutions announced yet another tentative agreement for a more formal affiliation. UCMC, renamed in 1979 as the University of Colorado Health Sciences Center (UCHSC), agreed to "move a major portion of its pediatric program to Children's and place the CU School of Medicine's principal teaching and research program at Children's." Administrators at both institutions downplayed opposition within the ranks, yet it persisted. Doctors at Children's still feared intrusions into their private practices. Other observers noted "a tug-of-war over which doctors from which hospital would get department chairs in the merger." A doctor at Children's assessed the conflict: "None of these guys want to give up a thing." Dr. Chang perceived a persistent problem in achieving affiliation on any long-term basis, stating, "What's important to CU doctors is research, not patient care."[6]

According to several veteran observers at Children's, a meaningful affiliation of numerous departments finally occurred in 1990, partly because economics dictated it. Merger had taken a long time, according to Children's Hospital board member Walter Rosenberry, in part because UCHSC negotiators "came to the table with a long spoon." In addition, he noted, key players in the negotiations kept changing. Yet realities slowly changed. By the mid-1980s pediatric services at University Hospital were dwindling, as local and regional competition became more intense. In contrast Children's was improving its clinical performance and financial base. Although some strong personalities at both institutions continued to resist, level-headed negotiators realized that affiliation was best for most concerned. Mr. Joseph H. Silversmith, Jr., president of the board of directors at Children's, toured many of the leading children's hospitals in the nation and learned that all of the leading institutions had affiliations with major university hospitals. Supporters emphasized that affiliation would also

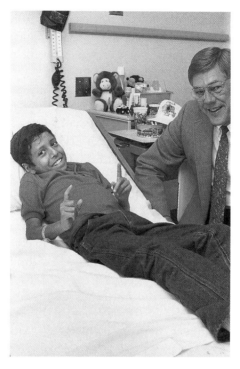

Dr. David G. Tubergen, director of oncology, later
to become medical director, visiting with a patient in the Oncology Center.

serve Children's interests. According to Dr. David Tubergen, former director of the Oncology Center and medical director at Children's in the late
1970s, merger brought more advantages than disadvantages. Expertise
expanded in many areas, and residents received far better training. Children's received the benefit of more advanced knowledge in pulmonary
medicine and liver and kidney transplants. A handful of strong individuals
left Children's because they opposed the affiliation, and the added numbers of patients caused some confusion, but by the early 1990s most
perceived it in positive terms.[7]

Although some doctors at Children's still reacted defensively when
research was on the agenda, the 1970s and 1980s marked great leaps
forward. Children's had contributed to the advancement in medical knowledge for several decades, primarily since the years of Dr. Harold D. Palmer.

Research efforts quickened after creation of the Oncology Unit in the mid-1960s.

Not surprisingly, the beginnings were modest. Several doctors received small local grants for research efforts in the 1960s. A major breakthrough occurred in 1972, when Drs. Blaise Favara and Charlene Holton obtained a $500,000 grant from the National Cancer Institute. In addition to funding their ongoing research, the NCI grant enabled them to create a Pathology Research and Training Center. In 1976 Children's Hospital built its first dedicated research laboratory, partly to attract Dr. Tubergen, who became director of pediatric oncology. In the mid-1970s several doctors set up research protocols in varying aspects of infectious diseases. Drs. Mimi Glode and George Pappas conducted their studies in a large warehouse facility on the northeast corner of the hospital's property. In 1978 Dr. James Todd and several associates described the toxic shock syndrome, associated with women's use of tampons. The latter discovery in particular brought considerable attention to research at Children's.

Despite these breakthroughs by dedicated individuals, Children's lost some research-oriented doctors who believed that institutional commitments to advancing medical knowledge were insufficient. In response Drs. Favara, Todd, and Jules Amer organized the Center for Investigative Pediatrics in 1978. In December of that year the Medical Executive Committee at Children's Hospital approved use of a $100,000 matching grant from the Piton Foundation to create an internal council to sponsor research. Piton Foundation support was largely the result of active promotion of Children's initiatives by Sam and Nancy Gary. The Center for Investigative Pediatrics, headed by Dr. Todd, provided seed money for projects that might attract outside funding. This strategy encouraged research-oriented doctors to compete for national-level awards. Dr. Ed McCabe received a major award from the Muscular Dystrophy Foundation for research on energy metabolism in muscle. Another group of investigators obtained a $1.5 million grant from the National Institutes of Health to explore Reyes syndrome therapy, and Dr. Mimi Glode received major private industry support for bacterial research.[8]

In the 1980s progress of research activity at Children's Hospital continued, but slowly. In August 1980 the C. Henry Kempe Center for Investigative Pediatrics was created as an outgrowth of the research center founded in late 1978. Named for the distinguished former chairman for pediatrics at UCMC who achieved important breakthroughs in infectious

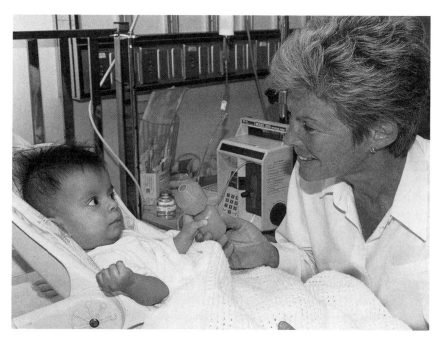

Nancy Gary, member of the board of directors, who with her husband Sam has funded and promoted pediatric research initiatives through the Piton Foundation.

diseases and child abuse and neglect, the center provided modern facilities for research-oriented doctors at Children's. Completed in 1981, thanks in part to a $330,000 Piton Foundation grant, the Kempe Center occupied the fourth floor of the Oca Cushman Wing. (This should not be confused with the Kempe National Center for the Prevention and Treatment of Child Abuse, a wholly separate organization.)

According to Dr. Todd, research at Children's still took a back seat to issues involving affiliation with UCHSC in the early 1980s. In May 1985, however, the Children's Hospital Foundation committed $200,000 per year in seed money for research in all departments. In the fall of 1985 Children's inaugurated its own journal, the *Quarterly Review*. Editor James W. Lustig, M.D., acknowledged that some might perceive its appearance as mere window dressing, designed to enhance the hospital's image: "One might wonder if the world needs another journal." Yet he argued that "there are

few publications which concentrate on promoting dialogue among physicians in practice and discuss state of the art treatment."[9] For practical
reasons the journal was short-lived.

In fact, research at Children's Hospital was oriented more toward
practical medicine than pure theory. As one early report from the Kempe
Center noted, "Local and national recognition is a key to generating funding for ongoing research and has a positive effect upon the institution's
image. But most importantly, an active and successful research program at
the Children's Hospital ensures each patient the availability of the most
advanced pediatric health care practices." In the late 1980s a number of
projects supported by the Kempe Research Center stressed the practical. A
major commitment to nursing research was made with the appointment of
Dr. Maureen Keefe (Ph.D.) of the Division of Nursing as associate director
of the center; she developed a nursing research program that became a
national model. In addition, research in sleep disorders commenced under
her direction. In 1988 the Kids Helping Kids Program was created. This
provided opportunities for high school and college students interested in
medical careers to work directly with researchers at the hospital.[10] Academic achievements also advanced careers at Children's. External funding
and publications in professional journals led to promotions. Internal funding by the Kempe Center leaped from $15,000 in 1985 to almost $1 million
in 1990. Publications by doctors and staff members numbered about fifty
each year in the late 1970s, and more than 150 per year in the late 1980s.[11]

Controversy at Children's Hospital over applied versus theoretical
research reflected national trends in the 1970s and 1980s. The 1970s marked
a resurgence of general and family practice, as well as continued differen-
tiation in ambulatory services available. The Society for Behavioral Pediatrics (SBP) was founded in 1982. Sensitive observers noted profound
changes in "children's" medicine by the 1980s. One historian observed,
"Increasingly, pediatricians are asked to support parents and children in
facing up to the psychological and environmental challenges of modern
society . . . [which] grow more onerous with each passing year."[12] These
included societal diseases such as divorce, child abuse, incest, "latch-key"
children, suicide, depression, AIDS, and various forms of substance abuse,
in addition to more familiar problems such as sexually transmitted diseases
and teenage pregnancies. However, as pediatric subspecialists multiplied,
they found themselves increasingly competing with specialists outside
pediatrics: child psychologists, special educators, social workers, and oth-

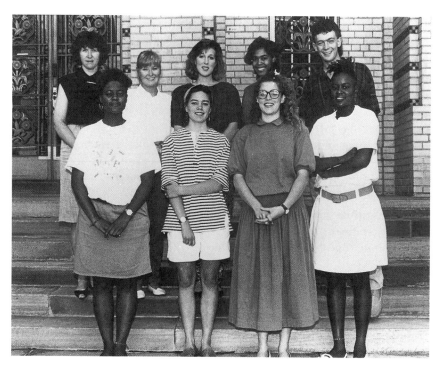

"Kids Helping Kids," a program for high school and college students interested in medical careers to work directly with researchers at Children's.

ers. No wonder many parents experienced confusion in determining how to deal with disturbed children and where to turn for professional help.

Growing complexity in service options available to bewildered parents reflected in part the unprecedented changes in the pediatric profession. Some highly skilled community pediatricians, like Dr. Jules Amer, remembered the procedures used in the 1950s when doctors admitted sick or injured children to Children's. After arranging admission to the hospital, these doctors then actively participated in providing appropriate therapy for "their" patients. By the early 1990s some general practitioners and pediatricians often felt displaced and complained that once they referred patients to Children's Hospital, they lost authority; the young patients were no longer "theirs." Even Amer, an experienced and respected practitioner, occasionally felt left out in referring patients.[13]

Dr. Seymour Wheelock recalled lengthy discussions within hospital walls and between paid staff at Children's and community physicians over how to resolve such issues. In Wheelock's view the primary issue was to avoid making Children's a high-tech–oriented institution: too cold, "efficient," or impersonal, in contrast to its time-honored role in providing nurturing pediatric care — care in which the office-based physicians continued to have an intimate, definitive role.[14]

Regional competition for patients continued to challenge leaders at Children's. By the mid-1970s, however, the hospital's reputation was solidly established. More than 100 hospitals in an eleven-state area referred patients needing acute care, which they could not provide, to Children's Hospital. The hospital's reputation as perhaps the premier children's facility in a multistate region was further enhanced by a variety of ancillary "arms" such as the Transport Service and a number of units (perhaps most notably the Burn Unit and the Newborn Center), which were supplied with the most sophisticated high-tech equipment available and staffed by nationally renowned specialists. Children's Hospital served many of the most critically ill patients within a 500,000-square-mile region. In 1976, for example, the hospital admitted 7,203 patients; 553 of these youngsters were from other states. Wyoming led with 157 admissions, followed by Kansas with ninety-five, New Mexico with thirty-four, South Dakota, twenty-nine, and Texas, twenty-two.[15]

The hospital was clearly excelling in terms of the type of health care delivered. In earlier years its programs emphasized the physical well-being of children. Like other successful hospitals around the country, Children's responded to new challenges in health care. In 1978 the hospital set up a Child Advocacy Team to deal with suspected child abuse, plus a Family Therapy Program. The latter unit assisted both victims and perpetrators of incest. The SIDS (sudden infant death syndrome) Counseling Center undertook the critical challenge of providing counseling for parents and families devastated by the unexpected loss of an apparently healthy child.[16]

Children's Hospital continued changing in response to demand. In the early 1980s it was clear that some children needed long-term care, including rehabilitation that employed specially trained staff and the latest in medical technology. As one of the select few facilities in the United States qualified to provide care to children with complex injuries, young patients were being referred from all over the country for rehabilitation services. Under the direction of Robert Bechtel, president, David Tubergen, M.D., senior vice president, and Beth Gaffney, associate director of planning, the Children's Hospital Rehabilitation Department was established by Jean McMahon, M.D., director of the Rehabilitation Diagnostic Clinic, Ann Grady, director of Occupational Therapy, and Lou Shannon, director of Physical Therapy; Dennis Matthews, M.D., was subsequently appointed chairman of the Department of Rehabilitation Medicine. The department quickly achieved national recognition in the treatment of children with spinal cord injuries, traumatic head injuries, orthopaedic injuries and brain damage from birth trauma, and many other conditions requiring rehabilitation.

Children's favorable competitive position was also enhanced by its willingness to coordinate services with other hospitals. For example, in 1978 the hospital entered into a joint venture with nearby St. Luke's to develop a comprehensive perinatal program. Dr. Butterfield, who negotiated the unique plan with the obstetricians at St. Luke's, appointed Dr. Peter Honeyfield to direct the program. St. Luke's had ample space; Children's had expertise to contribute. In a unique arrangement developed over many months of negotiations, Children's assumed all newborn services at St. Luke's. By such cooperative arrangements with other hospitals, Children's slowly expanded the number of its available beds in the late 1970s and 1980s. From a bed capacity of 157 in 1975 Children's expanded to 239 by 1990; almost all were a result of cooperative ventures with other institutions in east Denver's hospital zone and the emergence of specialized "off-site" nurseries.[17]

Results were gratifying, and statistics reflected an operation that was healthy in many ways. Although the hospital emphasized outpatient services, the number of inpatients did increase from 7,471 in 1975 to 9,251 in 1989. Outpatient visits increased more dramatically from just under 90,000 to almost 145,000 over the same period.[18]

Outpatient services frequently combined with new outreach programs in the 1980s. The Children's Hospital Home Care Program, initiated in 1983, was the brainchild of the internal staff, external health care professionals, and insurers. Newly available technology allowed for continued care for children at home, thus reducing hospital stays. Children with a wide variety of long-term medical needs have benefited. In 1984, its first full year of operation, program nurses made 752 visits and provided 1,142 treatments during 16,728 hours of work. By 1990 the figures were 4,052 visits and 4,696 treatments, spread over 40,001 hours.[19]

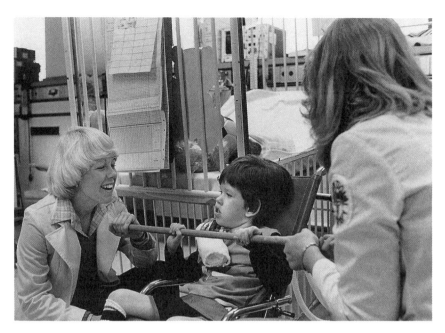

Billy Parkin, shown here with Terri Oberg-Carry, physical therapist, was a resident patient at Children's for the first five years of his life because of a rare, genetic muscle disease that allowed him to breathe only with the help of a respirator. Through support from staff, advanced technology, and the Home Health Care Program, Billy has been able to live at home and attend school. Photo by Michael Gamer.

In a parallel effort to better serve the metropolitan area through outreach, hospital leaders extended Children's presence to other parts of the region. In December 1986 Rehabilitation Services joined with the Department of Audiology and Speech Pathology and the Department of Behavioral Sciences to open the first Children's Hospital satellite at Hampden and Tamarac in southeast Denver. A second center was opened at Eightieth and Wadsworth in 1987, followed by a third center in Littleton in 1989.[20]

Numerical increases in patients served created still other challenges to leaders at Children's Hospital. During its first sixty-five years most new construction had occurred on a piecemeal basis. The hospital inevitably was an architectural hodgepodge, a combination of outdated and modern

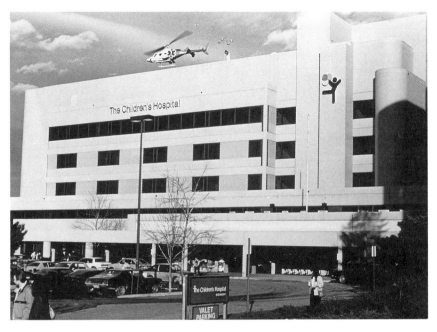

Five-story expansion of inpatient hospital facilities completed in 1979.

facilities. Although there was limited need for expanded bed capacity at Children's Hospital itself, modern medical practice required more space per bed. In order to provide a more attractive, modern, nurturing environment, hospital leaders had to tear down or renovate old space, as well as build new facilities.

Other worrisome realities confronted hospital decision makers. By the late 1970s inflation was rampant, and the consumer price index was rising at double-digit rates. For many reasons medical costs were even further out of control. Consequently leaders at Children's confronted a double-barreled challenge: modernizing and expanding facilities in the face of runaway costs. Their dilemma was exacerbated by the fact that because of negotiations with UCHSC administrators over the possible merger they had postponed modernizing and expansion.

Merger delays in the mid-1970s forced Children's leaders to deal with existing facilities. In the spring of 1976 the directors hired Kaplan,

McLaughlin Architects of San Francisco to create a future development plan at the present site. Although space was cramped, there was room for imaginative expansion. The designers recommended an addition adjacent to the north side of the Oca Cushman Wing. Most of the space would accommodate thirty-two intensive care and eighty acute care beds. The first floor would feature admitting offices, a pharmacy, an emergency entrance, and other services requiring immediate access. Completed in 1979 as a five-story facility, the new Health Center cost $8.3 million. Equally prescient, the designers foresaw additional expansion as far north as Twentieth Avenue in the late 1980s.[21]

These impressive gains were achieved despite daunting financial challenges. In retrospect it appears almost miraculous that Children's Hospital has operated in the black during most of its existence. As far back as World War I, hospital administrators worried about inflation and whether rising costs would prevent the hospital from delivering its services to all who needed them. Seventy years later, although dollar figures featured several more zeros, leaders at Children's wrestled with identical concerns. The institution prided itself on keeping its doors open to *any* child, no matter how poor the parents. However, during the first six months of 1980 uncompensated costs totaled $3.8 million. On August 21, 1980, the board of directors sadly announced that it would have to rescind the open-door policy. Henceforth some patients unable to pay would have to be referred elsewhere. Board president Jeaneene Anderson tried to soften the blow: "This policy certainly does not mean Children's will refuse or turn away emergency cases, which have no other place to be treated. . . . It is a policy whereby the hospital can screen and identify indigent referral cases in order to divert them safely to a public hospital or health care facility."[22] For many longtime associates and friends, the announcement marked the gloomiest day in the institution's history.

Yet given the financial realities of the time, leaders at Children's had little choice. A number of factors were driving health care costs through the roof. Children needing specialized treatment required more care at greater expense than adult patients; pediatric units in most general hospitals lost money. As the premier tertiary, or most intensive care hospital in the region, Children's received the majority of patients requiring treatments too complicated or specialized to be done at other nearby hospitals. In the late 1970s, 40 percent of the inpatients at Children's Hospital required intensive care, four times the rate for patients at general hospitals. As one analyst noted, "No pediatric hospital can survive on a steady stream of tertiary care patients. The cost of treating an intensive care patient is simply too high to expect full reimbursement."[23]

Reimbursement had become a major obstacle to administrators attempting to balance the books at U.S. hospitals. Even middle-class patients from families covered by solid insurance plans often caused losses. One problem was that insurers and hospital administrators had worked out long-term contracts, with fixed fees established for individual procedures. Theoretically an efficient administrative procedure, the policy had two weaknesses. First, the late 1970s medical costs were rising so fast that negotiated fees more than a few months old were outdated and inadequate. Second, medical science was advancing so rapidly that the medical-surgical staffs wished to introduce new procedures for which fees had not yet been negotiated. The latter challenge added mountains of paperwork and bureaucratic headaches.

An inkling of the financial problems facing Children's Hospital in recent years is found in the 1977 annual report. With a touch of nostalgia the writer noted that when the hospital was opened in 1910, the average cost per patient day was $1.46 and the average stay was 24.5 days. Sixty-seven years later the average length of stay had been cut to six days, but each day cost $297, still only a fraction of the $1,803 it cost in 1993. Equally ominous, the report noted that "charity, uncollectables, and contractual write-offs" had increased from $1.86 million to $2.8 million between 1976 and 1977.[24]

Hospital administrators were keenly aware that rapidly rising costs were not only bad for patients but damaging to the hospital's image. A significant portion of advertising budgets in the late 1970s was devoted to explaining rising costs to the public and describing steps Children's was implementing to fight inflation. Advertisements also stressed the enormous scientific and technological advances in medicine, particularly since World War II. In addition, they pointed out that medical care for children was particularly labor-intensive, requiring highly skilled caretakers, and labor costs had escalated rapidly. With the proliferation of high-tech equipment, numbers of specialists had to be on hand to attend the needs of a single patient. For example, to maintain the life of a two-pound premature infant, the Newborn Center might require the services of more than a dozen highly trained specialists: a respiratory therapist, radiologist, cardiologist, pulmonary consultant, neurosurgeon, ENT specialist, cardiovascular surgeon, gastroenterologist, general surgeon, pharmacist, social worker, and nurses, plus general housekeeping personnel. The mounting expense of providing heroic tertiary care was already evident in the late 1970s, and it would become an even more complex conundrum in the next decade.[25]

Other negative factors included increasing government regulation, the rapidly escalating costs of malpractice insurance, and increasing demand for services by health-conscious Americans who previously would have ignored medical treatment. A 1979 advertisement squarely placed Children's on the consumer's side: "We know you are concerned with the high cost of health care, and so are we." The same advertisement claimed that in 1978, costs to patients at Children's Hospital had climbed only 5.2 percent, "a figure substantially less than the national inflation rate."[26]

However valiant, cost-containment efforts were ineffective. Two years later Children's Hospital reluctantly resorted to its policy of "diverting" some indigent care patients. Even this failed to slow down rising costs. The 1980 annual report noted that in the final months of 1980, some twenty-five children were diverted safely to other institutions. Nevertheless, even after adjusting for inflation, Children's experienced a 35 percent increase over 1979 in losses from medically indigent patients.[27] Sadly the loss had increased nearly 400 percent in just five years.

A 1981 report noted that Colorado's population was well below the national average in age; fewer Coloradans were on Medicare, and typical hospital bills were below the national average. Ironically this may have worked to Children's Hospital's disadvantage, as higher proportions of the youthful regional population required subsidized services.[28]

Administrators at Children's made a concerted effort to battle rapidly escalating costs. One strategy involved lobbying the Colorado legislature on behalf of bills addressing their concern. In 1981 Dr. L. Joseph Butterfield, director of the Newborn Center, traced efforts of his staff since 1976 "to educate, recruit interest, and solicit funding for perinatal programs." He also noted that in 1981 House Bill 1301 "would provide a pilot program of health insurance, premium supplementation and catastrophic insurance." Butterfield urged his peers to "Pray for it. Better yet, engage in personal lobbying." Butterfield stated that shunting medically indigent patients to publicly funded hospitals was but one small example of "forestalling the wolf." He noted that in 1980 his unit had received 700 newborns from seventeen Denver and eighty-three regional hospitals, yet there was no policy for allocating costs. Children's simply absorbed charges that could not be collected. Butterfield advocated a more businesslike "bed-sharing" plan, wherein Children's would bill cooperating hospitals for services rendered. "In this concept, Children's becomes the partner of community hospitals without becoming the guarantor of payment — a munificence we cannot afford."[29] Butterfield compared the concept to time-sharing of any other facility.

Attempts to control costs at Children's were marginally effective at best. Responsible officials understood that many factors were beyond their control. They vacillated between accepting higher costs with philosophical resignation and considering drastic countermeasures. In June 1981 executive director Robert W. Bechtel stated Children's case in a letter to the editor of the *Rocky Mountain News*. By accepting charity cases and treating Medicaid patients, the hospital provided a public service that should be underwritten by public agencies. Bechtel chided the Colorado legislature for failing to enact a state catastrophic illness insurance program: "Our legislatures agree that rising hospital costs must stop and they agree on the severity of the medically indigent problem, but they can't agree on at least this one solution that would help slow the rate of increase."[30] As the numbers of medically indigent patients rose, costs had to be shifted to those who could pay. How much longer could even middle-class families absorb rising costs? That this problem was coming increasingly close to home was suggested by Dr. Jules Amer, who remembered a morning when a fourth-year medical student and his wife, a registered nurse, brought in their dehydrated six-month-old infant: "What came up during the ER visit . . . was that this poor, poor couple had no insurance — absolutely — and so I was told that the patient had to be hospitalized — [but] it couldn't be here [at Children's Hospital]. . . . I think we're all going to be medically indigent with spiralling costs."[31]

In June 1982 the board seriously proposed discontinuing contractual obligations to provide services under Medicaid and other government programs unless costs could be renegotiated on a more realistic basis. Three years later the director established a quota, a "bed allocation system" for patients unable to pay. Emergency cases would still be accepted, but outside physicians desiring to refer indigent patients were informed that admission would depend upon the availability of space.[32]

But none of these policies curbed uncompensated care costs. The 1980s marked a surge in uncollected fees. In 1981 the hospital billed $52.7 million and failed to collect $6.8 million. By the end of the decade billings

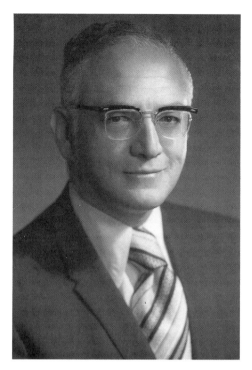

Joseph H. Silversmith, Jr., who served as treasurer and president of the board of directors, was elected first president of The Children's Hospital Foundation founded in 1980. Photo by Berkeley-Lainson-Denver.

had increased to $118 million, but uncompensated care had ballooned to $27.5 million, almost one-fourth of services billed. Without question these figures were exacerbated by double-digit annual rises in medical costs, and it was clear that the hospital was subject to many forces beyond its control.

In the early years leaders at Children's had successfully tapped the private sector for relief. Fund-raisers often put them over the top in allowing them to proceed with building projects. By the end of the 1980s such expectations had long since vanished. Hospital leaders repeatedly praised the generosity and public spiritedness of Denverites, but it was generosity of a different type: time. Unquestionably, volunteer activities were vital to the organization; in 1989 volunteers provided nearly 102,000 hours of service. Donations totaled $3.7 million, about 3 percent of expenses.[33]

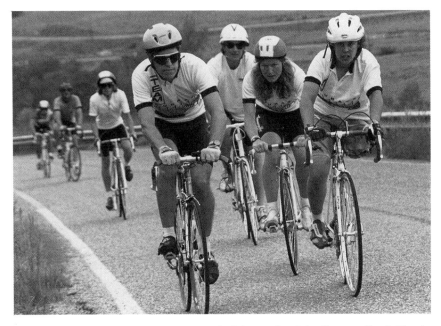

"Team Courage" member, Adrienne Rivera (right), completed the Courage Classic Bicycle Race with her trainers, including former Tour de France winner Marianne Martin (second from right).

By the early 1990s The Children's Hospital Foundation, formally established in November 1978, had evolved into a highly sophisticated, professionalized, independent unit. By skillful management of estate gifts and securities investments, plus a variety of community fund-raisers and other initiatives, the foundation provided total net revenues of nearly $8.7 million in 1992.[34]

The crisis atmosphere in health care during the 1980s forced Children's leaders to assess external influences, performance levels of hospital employees, and their own activities. Again they hired external consultants, this time M. Bostin Associates of New York. After lengthy review the consultants determined that the corporate structure was old-fashioned and inflexible. In March 1982 the board voted for a total reorganization of the hospital. Board president Joseph H. Silversmith, Jr., recalled that one reason for reorganization was that the hospital was earning money by the late

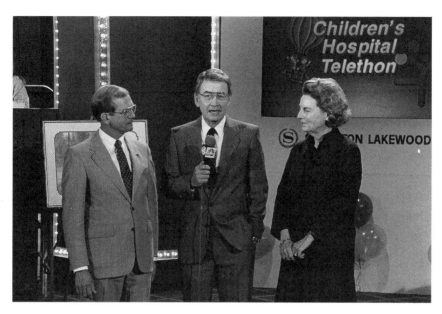

Bob Palmer, local television news anchor for KCNC (center), served as emcee for seven telethons. He is pictured here at the 1988 telethon with Lua R. Blankenship, Jr., president, and Frances N. "Salty" Welborn, chair, The Children's Hospital.

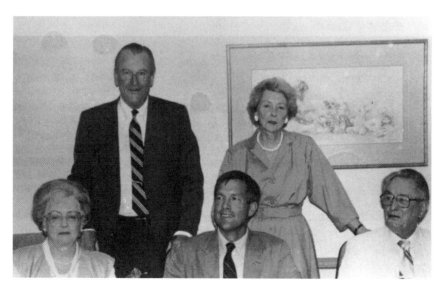

Mr. and Mrs. Don Vestal pictured here with Jeff Welborn, chairman of The Children's Hospital Foundation, and Mr. and Mrs. Calvin Fulenwider, Jr. The hospital named the sixth floor the Vestal Education Center in honor of the Vestals, who have donated over $5 million to fund programs at Children's. Both Peggy Fulenwider, a past president of the board of directors, and her husband Cal have been associated with the hospital for more than thirty-five years in numerous fund-raising activities.

1970s; separate entities would make the hospital better situated when seeking external funding. Second, dividing into several corporations would protect the hospital from catastrophic losses in the event of a lawsuit and would encourage funding, particularly federal grants. Health care delivery entailed greater risks than ever before by the early 1980s. Hospital president Robert W. Bechtel thought it prudent to spread them around.[35]

Rocky Mountain Child Health Services (RMCHS) was established under the new structure as a holding company to coordinate the activities of several subsidiaries. This included setting policies and guidelines for each affiliate's business activities, as well as coordinating and planning their programs. The holding company would monitor the activities of eight affiliated organizations and two subsidiary corporations. The affiliated organizations were: The Children's Hospital Association; Child Health Management Services, Inc.; Children's Emergency Transport Services, Inc.; Children's Hospital Foundation; Sewall Rehabilitation Center; Child Health Education Services, Inc.; The C. Henry Kempe Center for Investigative Pediatrics; Child Health Resources, Inc.; and R.M.I. The two subsidiaries were Early Horizons Child Care, Inc., and RMCHS Management Services, Inc.[36]

Executive Director Bechtel and his predecessor, Francisco Sabichi, symbolized a new breed of hospital administrators — concerned with patients but at the same time concentrating on the financial viability of the whole hospital organization. Bechtel's concentration on the financial health of the hospital continued throughout his service at Children's Hospital. This focus remained his top priority as the hospital embarked on a major building program. Although formal affiliation with UCMC did not occur until after Sabichi and Bechtel had left the organization, their efforts helped establish the groundwork to achieve that objective. The two men also recognized the importance of involving the medical and nursing staffs in making decisions with regard to clinical care. They were instrumental in establishing relationships with other hospitals in the area in an effort to consolidate pediatric care and thus reduce costs.

Reorganization of the hospital also occurred under Bechtel. Bechtel became president of the parent company. He was succeeded as president of the hospital by Lua R. Blankenship, Jr., who assumed that position in July 1983. Blankenship and his staff acknowledged that external challenges nearly overwhelmed even the soundest medical organizations in the early 1980s. Yet Silversmith recalled that many associated with Children's were

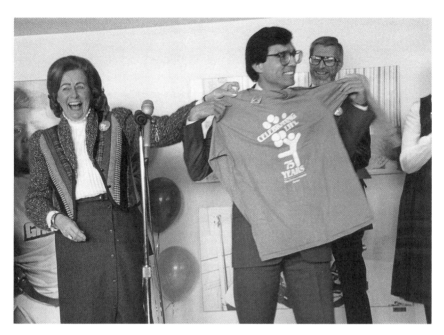

"Celebrating Life," the motto for the seventy-fifth anniversary. Shown here are Jeaneene F. Anderson, president of the board of directors, and Robert W. Bechtel, executive director, presenting Denver mayor Federico Peña a commemorative T-shirt.

quickly disillusioned with reorganization. "Our mistake was in bringing in administrative types rather than entrepreneurial types." He believed that the reorganization took place too quickly and with insufficient considera-tion of long-range objectives. "Most of the subsidiaries were great in theory and looked good on paper; but they never got off the ground." Dr. David G. Tubergen, medical director for most of the 1980s, was also unimpressed with the long-term outcomes from the reorganization. He agreed with Silversmith that few of the subsidiaries lived up to expectations. According to Tubergen some good people staked their professional reputations on them, and disagreements over their roles induced some dedicated people to leave Children's Hospital in the 1980s.[37]

Hospital leaders sensed that even with corporate reorganization the hospital's affairs were not running as smoothly as they should be. For the second time in two years they turned to M. Bostin Associates to assess its building program and future needs and the performance of the board of directors themselves.

In November 1983 the consultants delivered an assessment of the directors' activities that, despite polite language, was unflattering. In a nutshell, the board was too large, with too many persons who enjoyed the prestige of membership but did little or no real work. Some had been directors for years and had spotty attendance records at meetings. They remained board members, the consultants intimated, because nobody had summoned the courage to ask them to resign. Silversmith, the board president, believed that board members needed to be more businesslike, that far too much time was consumed with nonessentials, such as the best color for rooms and how long window drapes should be. The board of directors also needed more input from minorities in the community, plus direct influence by physicians. Since seven of eighteen members had served more than ten years, the consultants recommended a reduction in size and more frequent rotation of old members off the board.[38]

As Children's neared the end of its first eighty years, its very existence seemed threatened by powerful outside forces. Some wondered if tertiary-oriented, private institutions had a future. Yet few who knew Children's from the inside doubted its durability. In the words of Frances W. Welborn, chair of the board of directors in 1989, "Through the decades, regardless of changes in the health care industry, Children's mission has remained constant: to create and foster an environment where physicians, nurses and other health professionals work together for the highest quality care for children and their families."[39]

Cynics might dismiss such words as "apple pie and motherhood," but such aphorisms often contain seminal truths. In fact, Children's thrived late in the twentieth century precisely because leaders kept the focus on service. Both youngsters and their families sensed something special as soon as they entered the hospital. The modern hospital of the 1990s was a far more attractive place than its ancient predecessor of eighty years earlier. Children and their parents saw toddlers in brightly colored hallways with animals and soothing outdoor scenes painted on the walls. However busy nurses, doctors, orderlies, and cafeteria workers might be, a casual observer would see them stop to pick up a child who had fallen down or speak a few encouraging words to a youngster practicing with her crutches. Hospital personnel cared not only for children but for parents as well. Realizing that having a child with a critical illness was both physically and psychologically draining, hospital leaders saw to it that parents were saved from as much stress as possible. Visiting hours were literally any time, and parents could spend nights sleeping in the same room as their children. When they needed a night's uninterrupted sleep for themselves, they could stay at the nearby Inn at Emerson that was owned by Children's Hospital.

The meaning of Children's was conveyed in different ways to different people, and hospital outreach efforts assumed many different forms. Grade school students who had never been to Children's might receive a classroom visit from Harry Bear, "a lovable, furry patient complete with cast, identification bracelet and hospital pajamas." Harry would talk about what it was like to be in a hospital. Since the Harry Bear Visitation Program was undertaken by trained volunteers in 1976, Harry has reassured more than 10,000 area youngsters that a hospital visit need not be a terrifying experience.[40] Volunteers and staff members made prodigious efforts to bring joy to young patients, and they truly outdid themselves during holidays. On many occasions, they poked fun at holiday traditions, and themselves.

Over eight decades thousands of volunteers donated hundreds of thousands of hours of unpaid service to Children's Hospital. Without their contributions the hospital would not exist, at least as the unique institution it is today. It is impossible to acknowledge all of their efforts, yet several volunteers epitomize their spirit of sharing.

Emily Selig was born in 1916 and raised in Denver. Educated at Skidmore College, she married Leon Selig in 1938 and began a life of service to others. Over the course of a half-century she donated time and expertise to approximately two dozen public and private agencies, but her most important commitment was to Children's Hospital, where she began serving in 1949. Some of her duties were among the most stressful imaginable. She served in the Newborn Center and sometimes held and comforted dying infants in their last hours. Often their grieving parents simply could not deal with the emotional pain of doing so. She also helped families of critically ill babies take care of their own physical needs, arranging for places for them to stay. No doubt she preferred knitting clothes for infants or bringing flowers to cheer the staff.

Another "institution" at Children's Hospital is Mrs. Elliott Stacey, still going strong as a volunteer at age ninety-one. After moving to Denver from New York in 1949, Elliott immediately plunged into volunteer work. She did important work with other regional organizations (most notably the

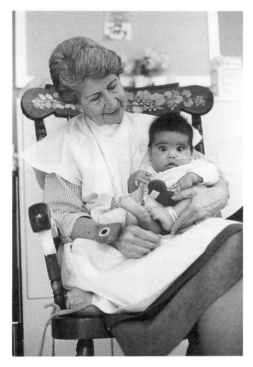

Emily Selig, a second-generation volunteer at Children's, comforting a young child who needed some special attention.

National Jewish Hospital), but her most significant contributions affected Children's Hospital. She joined the auxiliary in 1949 and served as president in 1952. Mrs. Stacey joined the board of directors in 1954 and held a number of important offices there, including a term as president in 1963. She concluded a quarter-century of work on the board in 1979 but was by no means just an executive. She did a considerable amount of hands-on, mundane work. To this day she can be found answering questions at the information desk or selling items at the thrift shop.[41]

Volunteers have expanded the scope of their activities since the mid-1970s. Fund-raising remains a key function, and two new ventures have been organized. The volunteers' thrift shop, Second Hand Annie's, opened its doors in the early 1980s. La Cache, a highly successful consignment shop inspired by volunteers Lenore Stoddart and Betsy Lewis and currently located at Fourth Avenue and Downing, began operations in

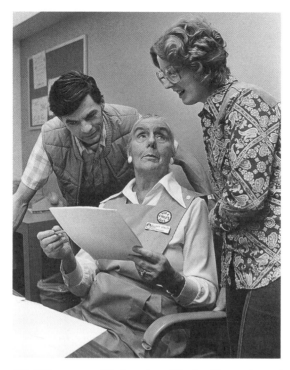

Elliott Stacey, one of the founders of the Auxiliary and a past president of the board of directors, shown here at the surgery desk providing information to family members on a patient's progress. Photo by Michael Gamer.

1982. In its first year La Cache sold $120,000 worth of goods and provided the hospital a profit of $35,000. Hundreds of volunteers discovered personal satisfaction in providing emotional support to the children. The Prescription Pet Program begun in 1986 brought joy to countless youngsters — and to the volunteers who witnessed small miracles occurring daily. The Handicapped Sports Program celebrated its twenty-fifth anniversary in 1993 and continues to work with the Winter Park National Sports Center for the Disabled. Today more than 150 children and their families participate in these year-round programs. As a result of this successful program, other children's hospitals have introduced their own versions.[42]

Young patients not yet well enough to participate in such strenuous activities continued to receive a constant stream of visitors, often unexpected. In addition to "prescription" puppies and exotic animals from the

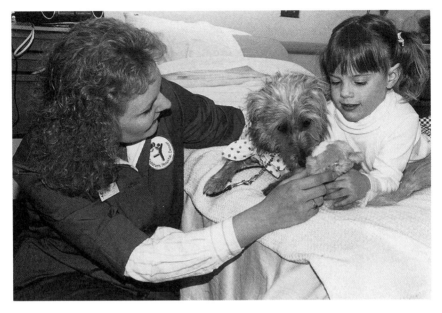

The Prescription Pet Program, co-founded by Janice Facinelli, D.V.M. (pictured here), and Fern Bechtel, director of volunteers, brings pets to divert and comfort the young patients. The program has won several national awards.

Denver Zoo, celebrity athletes from the Denver Broncos and Denver Nuggets, Mickey Mouse, the Cookie Monster from Shipsted and Johnson's Ice Follies, stars from the "Battlestar Galactica" TV show, Ronald McDonald, National Western Stock Show performers, Snoopy, and many other celebrities have brightened children's lives in recent years. Even the most severely handicapped children find reason for hope at Children's. By the early 1990s the hospital had acquired sophisticated personal computers that a quadriplegic child could operate by blowing or inhaling through a straw. This AccessAbility Resource Center Program, under the direction of Ann P. Grady, has attracted national attention; 2,000 children from six states received help in 1990.[43]

The end result of most of the hospital's ministrations was effective healing, sometimes bordering on the miraculous. In February 1989 three-year-old Kimberly Beesley was brought into the hospital by her frightened, bewildered parents. She had not responded to antibiotic drugs and was experiencing difficulty walking. To her parents' despair she was diagnosed

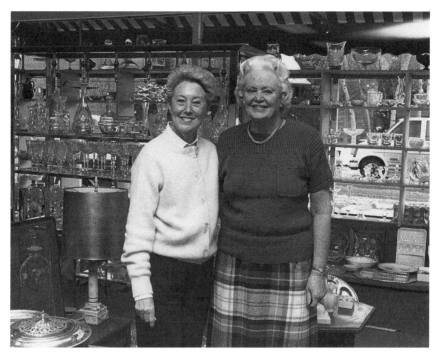

Pictured here are Betsy Lewis (left) and Lenore Stoddart, who organized a thrift shop and subsequently La Cache, a highly successful consignment shop, both staffed by volunteers, with proceeds used to fund activities at the hospital.

with childhood cancer, neuroblastoma. For several weeks, despite treatment, her condition appeared to worsen. Dr. Edward Arenson then sent her to UCLA where she "had her bone marrow harvested, purged and sustained a successful bone marrow transplant." A year after diagnosis, the tide had been turned, and her parents were ecstatic:

> I believe a miracle occurred for Kim, through medicine. No matter what happens to us in the future, Children's Hospital has stood firmly by us and together we've won the first battle. Children's is a very special place. The words "skilled," "professional," "love," "commitment" and "determination" come to mind. I will never forget Children's Hospital for giving us back a very special child.[44]

A Bone Marrow Unit was in full operation at Children's by 1994.

Other patients had similar experiences. Charley and Sandra Merrick of Sterling, Colorado, had a daughter in May 1987. The infant was diag-

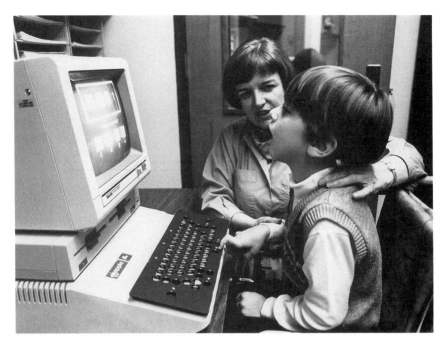

Ann Grady, past director of occupational therapy and seen here as director of the Children's AccessAbility Resource Program, teaching a patient to use highly sophisticated personal computers for fine motor coordination, learning communication, and leisure activities.

nosed as having hyperbilirubinemia and a heart murmur, as part of Down's syndrome. She was referred to Children's, where she had open-heart surgery to repair a ventricular-septal defect at age four months. Two years later she was fully recovered and, in her parents' words, "walking, talking and 'opening hearts' daily." They rhapsodized over their experience: "The atmosphere of 'one big family' at Children's was a tremendous help in relieving our anxiety. We were amazed and grateful for the quality of care Sarah received from *every* member of the hospital team."[45]

Patients remembered their experiences at Children's many years later, and many wrote to express their gratitude. Linda Pech of Northglenn, Colorado, recalled being admitted in 1977. At the time she was the shortest fifth grader in her class, by nearly a foot. Under Dr. Georgeanna Klingensmith's care, and with triweekly injections for hormone deficiency along with repeated follow-up visits over several years, she achieved a

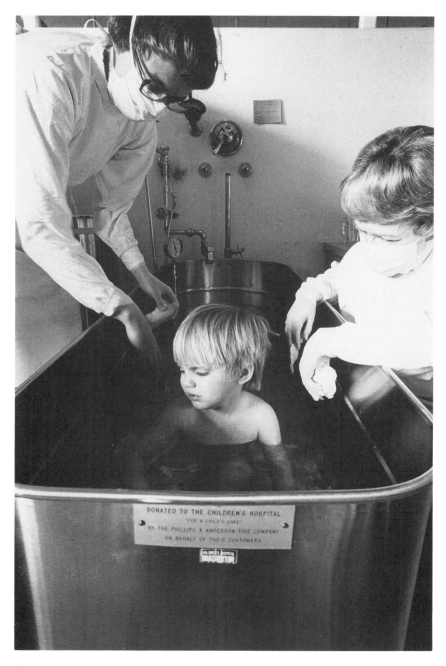

Burn patient receiving treatment from a nurse and therapist in a special whirlpool bath donated by the Phillips & Anderson Tire Company on behalf of their customers.

normal height: "My self-esteem grew with my stature and I will always be grateful to the nurses, doctors, patients and everybody else at Children's who made my treatment and future a success."[46] Even families whose children lost the struggle for survival often recalled their experiences at the hospital with gratitude. The Bailey family of Louisville, Colorado, lost their three-month-old son to nonaccidental trauma. They allowed their infant to become an organ donor: "Kevin couldn't have received better care, I'm convinced. In May of 1989 we came to the PCIU unit to talk about our feelings about organ transplantation . . . and, again, we were impressed with the care and concern people still had, more than a year after his death."[47]

Treatment provided to children in the late twentieth century differed markedly from that of eight decades earlier. In the early years, much of the emphasis was upon simple feeding and lengthy, if mundane, treatments for infants and young people. By the 1990s, of course, tens of thousands of routine outpatient services were performed each year. Children's was as committed to preventing sickness as to curing sick children. Many young persons came to Children's just once for a simple test or a routine operation requiring no overnight visit. Hospital personnel much preferred seeing healthy youngsters walk out of the hospital within hours or even minutes of arrival. Obviously, however, some inpatient treatments rendered were critical, delicate, "heroic" medical practices.

Although constituting only a small percentage of the total number of patients treated in a given year, the cases of dramatic procedures to save a child's life have grown steadily in recent years. The Newborn Center continued to perform dramatic rescue operations. Other units enjoyed similar success and worked equally impressive miracles. The Burn Team was established in 1974 under the enlightened leadership of Dr. William C. Bailey, and within a year it managed to save patients with burns over as much as 86 percent of their bodies. A thirteen-year-old girl named Endina from Olathe, Colorado, whose dress was ignited by an electric space heater, suffered burns over nearly half her body, and her chances of survival were only 50 percent when she was flown in. She stayed at Children's three months and underwent eight operations for removal of burned skin and replacement skin grafts. Her family was unable to visit often, so two volunteers "adopted" Endina and visited her every day. Many specialists were involved, as Endina needed far more than simply physical restructuring. Psychological counseling was provided to Endina and her family, and plastic surgeons, orthopaedists, occupational and physical therapists, and other experts were called in.[48]

Miranda Soper was fourteen in 1987. She suffered a traumatic head injury in an automobile accident in October and was brought to Children's, where she remained in a coma for three months. Regaining consciousness in January 1988, she spent the next three months in the Rehabilitation Unit. She was finally sent home in April, and her mother remembered her as being almost totally helpless: "It frightened me to see how dependent she was; she couldn't even feed herself." But Children's Hospital Home Care Program helped the family provide the right setting to encourage the patient to learn to do things on her own. In the words of one of the therapists, "In their own homes, during a time that's best for the family and child, children make progress you would never imagine, having seen them in the hospital." Her mother expressed her gratitude for the vision of therapists at the hospital: "I know that without the resources and therapists from Children's Hospital, Miranda wouldn't be home. I couldn't do without them, and I think I would have gone mad. The accident is something I will never accept. But with the help from the Children's Hospital, we are learning to live with it."[49]

These and countless other recent cases suggest how far Children's Hospital has come from the early years. Nevertheless, runaway medical costs and other sobering questions in the late twentieth-century United States have forced decision makers at Children's to deal with perplexing questions of medical ethics. A young mother delivered her baby son sixteen weeks prematurely. He weighed only 1.5 pounds at birth and spent his first seven months at the hospital on maximum support from technology and the staff at the Newborn Center. The cost was $375,000, which neither insurance nor the family covered. Hospital spokespersons noted that as little as $400 spent on prenatal care might have prevented the mother's premature delivery. They asked: "Can we afford the cost of survival without making prevention a priority?"[50] The constant expansion of outpatient clinics reflects the fact that Children's leaders have emphasized prevention for years, particularly since World War II.

Preventive medicine has been the foremost goal in pediatrics since founding of the specialty. By the late twentieth century practicing physicians had at their disposal technological assistance undreamed of a few decades earlier. To some observers, however, there is a negative aspect of rapid technological advances: they fear that too many doctors become so

C. Richard Hawes

Dr. Hawes is an "old-timer" in terms of service, yet his infectious enthusiasm for his patients and everything associated with Children's mirrors the exuberance of perpetual youth.

He grew up in Oklahoma and earned both his B.S. and M.D. degrees at the University of Oklahoma, the latter in 1946. Completing a rotating internship at the Gallinger Municipal (now D.C. General) Hospital in Washington, Hawes received training in obstetrics, gynecology, and syphilology. He was a member of the team that established the Romansky unit measurement of penicillin.

Following a stint with the army, he returned to Norman, Oklahoma, and set up a successful family practice. But his real interest was pediatrics, so he joined the staff at Children's Hospital in 1951. Within two years Hawes had married staff nurse Elsie Opsahl, his wife of forty years, and had volunteered to help build up the Cardiology Unit. An expert in congenital heart disease, he made numerous contributions to the development of new techniques for repairing defective hearts. Hawes also was called upon to spend increasing amounts of time administering various departments and units. He was assistant medical director from 1956 to 1961; in 1957 he became director of the Cardiopulmonary Laboratory, and in 1981 he became chief of cardiology.

Although periodically active in research, Hawes is most committed to teaching medical students and serving his patients. His warmth and encouragement have changed many young lives for the better. He is widely admired and loved by his patients and colleagues. In 1965 the *Denver Post* prematurely published his photo in an obituary column, but more than a quarter-century later he is still going strong, enjoying his hobbies of history, archaeology, and fly-fishing. Little wonder that he is almost always smiling.[51]

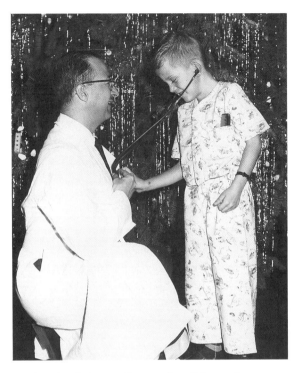

Dr. C. Richard Hawes, director of cardiology who came to
Children's as a resident in pediatrics in 1951, is shown here
with Jeff Stone.

enthralled by scientific advances that they lose touch with their patients as
human beings. An example is the emotional debate over "heroic" methods
for keeping premature infants alive. In newborn centers all across the
nation, as well as at Children's Hospital, highly sophisticated equipment
and advanced techniques combine to save some infants with birth weights
of barely over one pound. Despite solid evidence in the early 1990s that
growing percentages of seriously underweight babies are surviving and
that a small percentage have a decent prospect of becoming functioning
adults, serious ethical questions arise. Can we afford to keep them alive? If
not, who should make the decision to terminate life-support treatments?
Although much of the contemporary debate over escalating health costs
focuses on the elderly, many hospitals spend more for keeping tiny infants
alive on life-support equipment.

Doris J. Biester

In 1979 the director of nursing position was elevated to senior vice president, nursing director. Doris J. Biester, who had served as assistant director of nursing at Women's and Infant's Hospital in Rhode Island, joined the hospital staff, and with her arrival the status of the nurse at Children's changed.

In 1984 an all-professional nursing staff was implemented. No longer would Licensed Practical Nurses (L.P.N.s) and nurse's aides serve. All nurses hired were required to hold the Bachelor of Science in Nursing degree. A Professional Nurse Internship Program to support the new B.S.N. graduates in their transition from student to practicing pediatric professional was established. Although individual nurses had been involved in research, a Nursing Research Program was formalized in 1985. Family-centered care intensified and a change in dress code allowing nurses to wear street clothes was approved.

Doris Biester worked to strengthen and formalize collaborative relationships with the UCHSC School of Nursing, which served as a role model in later negotiations between the hospital and the Department of Pediatrics during merger discussions.

A recent in-depth story in the *New York Times* quoted doctors who insisted that if they could produce one healthy baby out of 100 very underweight babies, they had a moral obligation to do so. Critics observed that the vast majority of newborns under two pounds would suffer severe brain damage even if they lived. Too often physicians have allowed their professional egos to obscure humane consideration of both the infants' and their parents' interests. In some cases doctors have kept babies on life-support equipment against the wishes of distraught parents. Costs are horrendous: $2,000 a day, or up to $500,000 for four months.[52] Medical ethics committees must grapple more effectively with the moral and financial dilemmas associated with balancing runaway costs and compassion in applying "heroic" medicine.

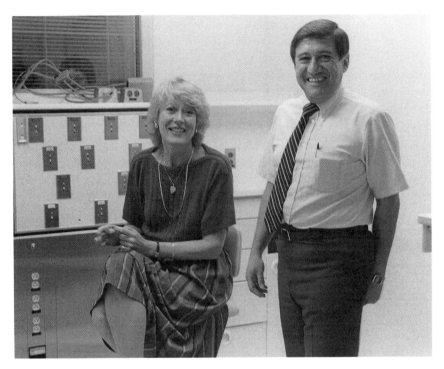

Doris Biester, R.N., M.S., F.A.A.N., senior vice president for Patient Care Services Administration, and Jacinto Hernandez, M.D., chief of neonatology, discussing patient care needs in the Newborn Center.

Such worrisome issues have concerned decision makers at Children's Hospital since its inception, but even more so in recent years. An annual report from the late 1980s stressed medical ethics. A responsible, hard-working, middle-aged couple in Denver owned their family business and had six children ranging in age from nine months to sixteen years. The family had very expensive coverage under a program for people with small businesses. Unfortunately that insurance company went out of business. The only coverage they could find cost between $800 and $1,000 per month, which they could not afford. The parents gambled on no coverage and lost. The mother became pregnant, and the baby was born with Down's syndrome. Although the family could care for the baby from savings over the short term, the long-term prognosis was for years of costly treatment. Who would pay? Dr. Jeff Scott of Children's Hospital noted, "We're coming to the breaking point concerning health care in our society. And it becomes especially clear when families like [this one] are without affordable health coverage for their children." Frustrated over the financial strain on a family whose son was undergoing long-term cancer treatment and who had experienced numerous debilitating and expensive setbacks, another doctor noted: "We need a national commitment that all children have equal access to health care. Like education, health care must be a child's right, not a privilege."[53]

As the 1990s opened, Children's Hospital clearly filled vital needs in specialized health care in the region. Inpatient admissions had grown somewhat in the 1980s. In 1990, 9,275 inpatients were admitted; they stayed an average of just over one week, and the hospital provided 66,248 days of care. Outpatient services continued to grow at a healthy pace, with 188,679 visits recorded. More than 1,000 doctors were on the combined medical and surgical staff, including 313 residents/interns. Employing 2,195 people, the hospital had a total 1990 payroll of $53.8 million. Patient revenues amounted to $144.9 million, but the uncompensated health care problem was just getting worse, amounting to $34.4 million in 1990 alone.[54] Financing health care remained a critical, unsolved problem as the new decade opened.

Although the annual report in 1989 focused on the more negative question, "How long can children remain on the critical list?", virtually all who knew Children's Hospital were inspired by the monumental goals it had achieved in its first eight decades. Health care for children in the Rocky Mountain region was not only vastly improved over that offered eighty years earlier, but Children's Hospital stood out in the national network of hospitals for children and the pediatric units of general hospitals. Children's Hospital made the benefits of stunning advances such as the Salk vaccine and other lifesaving scientific breakthroughs quickly available to children throughout a multistate region, and it achieved medical miracles with the assistance of gleaming technological innovations. Yet all who are intimately involved with the hospital realize that equally critical healing continues on a daily basis: in the warm, caring ministrations given by physicians, nurses, other hospital personnel, and volunteers. As smiles and laughter replace pain and tears, workers and volunteers witness the positive results of their efforts dozens of times each day. Certainly the founders of Children's Hospital could be proud of what they started.

Notes

1. *Bambino* (January 1978): 1. This is an internal newsletter published by Children's Hospital.

2. Harry P. Ward, M.D., to Francisco D. Sabichi, March 4, 1976; Dr. Thomas Starzl to Dr. Edward P. Duffie, May 20, 1976; both in CHD Collection.

3. Mayo and UPMS sources both quoted in Robert L. Telender to Mr. J. H. Silversmith, Jr., February 2, 1977, CHD Collection.

4. Ibid.; Jack Chang, M.D., to Richard Olmsted, M.D., July 21, 1978; Dr. Robert Hendee to Olmsted, July 26, 1978; both in CHD Collection.

5. Olmsted to William E. Hathaway, M.D., February 14, 1979; Minutes, Meeting of Critical Care Committee, January 23, 1979.

6. *Denver Business Journal*, February 20, 1989, 1, 22; Chang to Olmstead, July 21, 1978.

7. Walter S. Rosenberry III, taped interview by Winifred Moss, August 15, 1991; Dr. David G. Tubergen, taped interview by Winifred Moss, August 12, 1991; Joseph H. Silversmith, Jr., taped interview by Winifred Moss, May 19, 1991; all in CHD Collection.

8. James K. Todd, M.D., "Clinical Science With a Heart: The History of Research at The Children's Hospital, 1910–1990," 1991, Physician Typescript, CHD Collection, 6–7.

9. Ibid., 8; *Quarterly Review* 1 (Fall 1985): Foreword.

10. "The Children's Hospital Kempe Research Center," n.d., pamphlet published by Children's Hospital, CHD Collection.

11. Todd, "Clinical Science With a Heart," 9.

12. Sydney A. Halpern, *American Pediatrics: The Social Dynamics of Professionalism, 1880–1980* (Berkeley: University of California Press, 1988), 142–143, 145; Thomas A. Cone, M.D., *History of American Pediatrics* (Boston: Little, Brown and Co., 1979), 241.

13. Dr. Jules Amer, tape of presentation ca. 1985, CHD Collection.

14. Seymour Wheelock, M.D., informal interviews with Mark S. Foster, Summer 1993.

15. Children's Hospital advertisement, March 27, 1977; Robert W. Bechtel, "A Children's Hospital Moves to Embrace the Future," manuscript, ca. 1982, 1–2; both in CHD Collection.

16. *1978 Annual Report*.

17. "Celebrate," CHD pamphlet, ca. 1986, 17–18; *1975 Annual Report*; *1990 Annual Report*, 12.

18. *1975 Annual Report*; *1989 Annual Report*, 12.

19. "The Children's Hospital Home Care Program, 1983–1900," September 1993, manuscript, CHD Collection.

20. "History, Specialty Care Centers," 1993, manuscript, CHD Collection.

21. *A Development Plan: The Children's Hospital of Denver* (San Francisco: Kaplan, McLaughlin Architects, 1976), 7, 13, 20, 23, 47.

22. *Medical Staff News* (March 1981): 10.

23. "Our Commitment to Children," ca. 1979, mimeograph in CHD Collection, 4.

24. *1977 Annual Report*. Costs for patients per day continued to mount uncontrollably in the early 1990s: in 1990, $1,441; in 1991, $1,620; in 1992, $1,630. Figures provided by Lindy Schultz, executive assistant to Lua Blankenship, December 14, 1993.

25. Information from Winifred Moss in telephone conversation with Mark S. Foster, June 30, 1993.

26. Advertising supplement to the *Denver Post*, undated, 1979.

27. *1980 Annual Report*.

28. "Health Care in Colorado: A Matter of Facts," pamphlet (Denver: Colorado Hospital Association, 1981).

29. Ibid.

30. Robert W. Bechtel to Editor, *Rocky Mountain News*, June 4, 1981.

31. Amer, Oral interview.

32. "Cost Shift and Fund Allocation for Uncompensated Health Care," mimeograph, November 23, 1982; Charlie Hebeler to Members of the Board of Directors, July 11, 1985; all in CHD Collection.

33. *1981 Annual Report; 1985 Annual Report; 1989 Annual Report*, 12.

34. *1992 Annual Report*, 5.

35. Silversmith interview by Moss, May 19, 1991.

36. "Rocky Mountain Child Health Services, Inc.," November 1985, mimeograph in CHD Collection.

37. Silversmith interview by Moss, May 19, 1991; Tubergen interview by Moss, August 12, 1991.

38. M. Bostin Associates, "The Children's Hospital, Denver, Colorado: Assessment of the Board of Directors," draft report, November 1983; Silversmith interview, May 19, 1991.

39. *1989 Annual Report*, 1.

40. "Harry Bear and Friends," n.d., pamphlet, CHD Collection.

41. Kathleen McBride to Mark Foster, July 9, 1993, in possession of Foster.

42. *Impact* (Winter 1988): 2–7. This is one of CHD's internal publications.

43. "User Friendly," *Rocky Mountain News Sunday Magazine*, January 27, 1991.

44. Joan and Ed Beesley to Children's Hospital, November 1989, CHD Collection.

45. Sandra L. Merrick to Children's Hospital, October 1989, CHD Collection.

46. Linda Pech to Children's Hospital, ca. 1989, CHD Collection.

47. Cassi Bailey to Children's Hospital, ca. 1989, CHD Collection.

48. *1975 Annual Report*.

49. *1988 Annual Report*.

50. *1989 Annual Report*, 2.

51. *Bambino* (August/September 1981): 8–9.

52. *New York Times*, September 29, 30, October 1, 1991.

53. Jules Amer, M.D., tape of presentation, ca. 1989, 6–7, CHD Collection; *1989 Annual Report*, 5, 9.

54. *1990 Annual Report*, 12.

Postscript

If there is anything that stands out in reading this wonderful story of the first eighty years of The Children's Hospital of Denver, it is that *change is inevitable*. We have seen a health care institution that began as a tent clinic near City Park, now grown to a complex campus of buildings reflecting an evolving mission and ever-expanding technologic capabilities. From humble local roots we have expanded into a regional referral resource, facilitated by an increasingly sophisticated communication and transportation system. An initial focus on rehabilitation evolved, first to the successful treatment and now the prevention of many diseases that previously crippled the region's children.

The provision of basic clinical care has expanded to include quality improvement and clinical research; after years of negotiation and debate we now stand as the preeminent pediatric education and research institution in this area. We see our mission not just as a hospital but as a children's health care system, meeting the needs of children on an increasingly ambulatory basis, with prevention of disease the ultimate goal.

How different are the halls of the present Children's Hospital! The multiple buildings on our growing campus serve as architectural testimony to the changing emphasis of a responsive institution — as technology advanced, so did The Children's Hospital of Denver. Past diseases that occupied much of its early history have now been eliminated or controlled. Effective treatments for gastroenteritis, tuberculosis, osteomyelitis, and hyaline membrane diseases have been developed. Vaccines have virtually eradicated smallpox, polio, measles, pertussis, diphtheria, tetanus, rubella, mumps, and, most recently, *Hemophilus influenza* meningitis — all diseases that filled our wards and devastated children in the past. Modern diagnostic testing in the laboratory and imaging departments permits the early recognition and treatment of most diseases. Antibiotics — considered the greatest medical advance of the twentieth century — now treat not only bacteria but also fungal and even viral infections. Intravenous techniques permit the use of medical therapies and system support never before

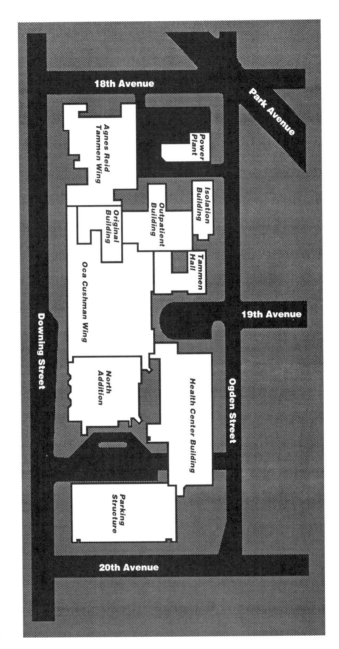

possible. A triumph of the past twenty years is the emergence of effective cancer chemotherapy, which has had its greatest success in treating children. Our neonatal and pediatric intensive care units are a far cry from the limited iron lung support that was available in the polio era. New pediatric surgical techniques have led to the palliation and cure of many previously fatal or incapacitating congenital and acquired diseases. The development of molecular genetic techniques offers the hope even now of preventing and curing many inherited diseases.

We cannot be complacent, as there are many challenges to be faced. As our children have become physically stronger and healthier, they have become more psychologically and socially stressed. Values have eroded. Society is fragmented. Violence abounds. Drug and other substance abuse in our children is on the increase. Our educational system is faltering, and our economy is struggling. New diseases like AIDS create new medical challenges.

And yet at Children's Hospital, amongst all these challenges and changes, some things have remained constant. We retain the greatest depth and breadth of pediatric expertise in the region. Our child-focused support services cannot be equaled. The team approach of pediatric professionals — nurses, pharmacists, primary-care physicians and specialists — that began in the early years with Dr. Minnie C.T. Love and Oca Cushman, has not changed. The tradition of volunteer and benefactor involvement in The Children's Hospital continues to remind us of the importance of our mission not only as a vocation but as an avocation as well. Equally important, we remain a focus of the training of most of the pediatric health care practitioners in the community, creating an ongoing partnership in the care of children in the region. Finally our commitment to the advancement of care through quality improvement and clinical research ensures our ability to respond to future challenges, creating "tomorrow's care today."

As we face the complexity of evolving health care reform in a competitive environment with limited resources and large, underserved populations, we must continue to embrace change. The Children's Hospital of Denver *has* evolved; it *has* responded to the challenges of the times. It is that ability to change — so clear from its history — that affirms its promise to meet the future needs of children. We remember the words of Max Ginsburg forty years ago: "Children's Hospital should not merely be a place where children get good treatment and services for their illnesses. . . . We must lead in the newer forms of therapy which only a specialized hospital can offer. . . . This institution should be a source of intellectual stimulation." If there is one conclusion we can draw from an awareness of the hospital's history, it is that change is not only inevitable, *change is desirable*. As The Children's Hospital recognizes and responds to the changing needs of children, it will continue to define and deliver the care of the future — for a child's sake.

James K. Todd, M.D.

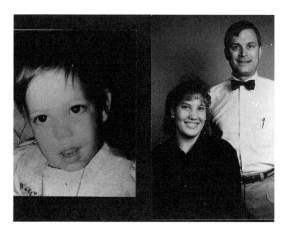

May 10, 1993

Dear Dr. Todd:

Enclosed is an invitation to my graduation from Lincoln High School in Des Moines, Iowa and my graduation picture. In 1975 I was a patient of yours. I was admitted to Children's Hospital on July 5, 1975 with Meningitis.

I just wanted you to know that I'm doing well and with your help I'm graduating!

Thank you for all you did for me.

Sincerely,

Melissa Krinn

Melissa Krinn, shown here in 1975 and again with Dr. James K. Todd in 1993, taken when she visited Dr. Todd at Children's after her high school graduation.

Appendix

THE CHILDREN'S HOSPITAL, Denver, Colorado, wishes to acknowledge the commitment and dedication of the following:

a. Presidents of The Children's Hospital Association
b. Presidents of the Medical Staff
c. Presidents of the Auxiliary of The Children's Hospital
d. Administrators
e. Medical Directors
f. Directors of Nursing

Presidents of The Children's Hospital Association

Mrs. E. A. Coburn
Mrs. Edward Wynne Williams
Mrs. James Williams
Mrs. William V. Hodges
Mrs. Thomas Keely
Mrs. William H. Kistler
Mrs. Lafayette M. Hughes
Mrs. Melville Black
Mrs. L. Kent Robinson
Mrs. Edward G. Knowles
Mrs. Henry C. Van Schaack
Mrs. Harry C. Brown
Mrs. Harry H. Tammen
Mrs. Dean Clark
Mrs. Van Holt Garrett
Mrs. Harry C. Brown
Mrs. Hector C. McNaught
Mrs. Walter W. Blood

Mrs. Van Holt Garrett
Mrs. E. Ray Campbell
Mrs. Arthur G. Rippey
Mrs. Edward G. Knowles
Mrs. Mason A. Lewis
Mrs. Raymond E. Sargeant
Mrs. Harry S. Silverstein, Jr.
Mrs. Emmett H. Heitler
Mrs. Wayne Stacey
Mrs. Darrell J. Hamilton
Mrs. L. Calvin Fulenwider, Jr.
Mrs. John T. Stoddart, Jr.
Lawrence R. Reno
Cyrus A. Hackstaff
Mrs. Norman Davis
Joseph H. Silversmith, Jr.
Terrence J. Ryan
Jeaneene F. Anderson

Title changed to Chairman

Virginia D. Skartvedt   Kathryn L. Powers
Walter S. Rosenberry III   Frances N. "Salty" Welborn
Oliver Hickel III   Larry J. Hauserman

Presidents of the Medical Staff

George B. Packard, Sr., M.D.   Ralph W. Danielson, M.D.
Franklin P. Gengenbach, M.D.   Mariana Gardner, M.D.
T. E. Carmody, M.D.   H. A. Buchtel, M.D.
John W. Amesse, M.D.   William D. Rothwell, M.D.
Robert G. Packard, M.D.   Douglas W. Macomber, M.D.
Emanuel Friedman, M.D.   Joseph H. Lyday, M.D.
Roy P. Forbes, M.D.   John M. Nelson, M.D.
H. W. Wilcox, M.D.   William F. Stanek, M.D.
G. M. Blickensderfer, M.D.   Seymour E. Wheelock, M.D.
George B. Packard, Jr., M.D.   Edward B. Plattner, M.D.
Wiley W. Jones, M.D.   James E. Strain, M.D.
William M. Bane, M.D.   Peter C. Hoch, M.D.
H. L. Baum, M.D.   Alvin P. Miller, M.D.
W. W. Barber, M.D.   Charles Brown, M.D.
Hamilton I. Barnard, M.D.   Edwin T. Williams, M.D.
F. B. Stephenson, M.D.   Leo J. Flax, M.D.
J. A. Schoonover, M.D.   Felice A. Garcia, M.D.
Rex L. Murphy, M.D.   F. Henry Reynolds, M.D.
Atha Thomas, M.D.   Jules Amer, M.D.
J. E. Russell, Jr., M.D.   William A. Campbell III, M.D.
Luman E. Daniels, M.D.   Lewis R. Day, M.D.
Harold L. Hickey, M.D.   L. Joseph Butterfield, M.D.
Louis C. Wollenweber, M.D.   Robert W. Hendee, Jr., M.D.
Roderick J. McDonald, Jr., M.D.   J. Darrell Miller, M.D.
Ralph H. Verploeg, M.D.   Robert E. Eilert, M.D.
Herman I. Laff, M.D.   Jerry W. Taylor, M.D.
William R. Lipscomb, M.D.   John B. Campbell, M.D.
Harry C. Hughes, M.D.   Edmund N. Orsini, Jr., M.D.
Max M. Ginsburg, M.D.   Paul N. Tschetter, M.D.
F. Craig Johnson, M.D.   John D. Strain, M.D.

Presidents of the Auxiliary of The Children's Hospital

Mrs. Warren Robinson
Mrs. Arthur Rydstrom
Mrs. Wayne Stacey
Mrs. G. R. Harris
Mrs. Kenneth Schmidt
Mrs. Ferris Ruggles
Mrs. George Liljestrom
Mrs. John Ambler
Mrs. Frank Devitt
Mrs. John Ryland
Mrs. Seth Bradley
Mrs. Joseph L. Boettner
Mrs. James Shannon
Mrs. John Tyler

Mrs. Leonard Sahlen
Mrs. John Macleod
Mrs. Robert Waterman
Miss Amy Davis
Mrs. Wayne Cavender
Mrs. Richard Kintzele
Mrs. Gordon Close
Mrs. William Dabney
Mrs. William Lewis
Mrs. Emmett Stephenson
Mrs. Robert Siegrist
Mrs. James Cohig
Mrs. Richard Schaefer
Ms. Linda Surbaugh

Administrators

Oca Cushman, R.N.
Robert B. Witham
DeMoss Taliaferro
Norman L. Losh

Francisco D. Sabichi
Robert W. Bechtel
Lua R. Blankenship, Jr.

Medical Directors

Harold D. Palmer, M.D.
John R. Connell, M.D.

Merl J. Carson, M.D.
Frank J. Cozzetto, M.D.

Acting Medical Director

L. Joseph Butterfield, M.D.

Edward R. Duffie, M.D.

Interim Medical Director

Max Kaplan, M.D.

Acting Medical Director

Seymour E. Wheelock, M.D.   David G. Tubergen, M.D.
Richard W. Olmsted, M.D.   Peter L. Durante, M.D., J.D.*

Directors of Nursing

E. Luella Morrison, R.N.   Alice Alcott, R.N., B.S.
Joy Erwin, R.N., M.A.   Sylvia G. Hoover, R.N., B.A., M.A.
Ada Koebke, R.N., B.S.   Margaret Greczyn, R.N.
Inez L. Armstrong, R.N., M.S.   Doris J. Biester, R.N., M.S., F.A.A.N.

---

*Position title changed to Director of Medical Affairs

Index